Medicine: The Forgotten Art?

Christopher Elliott-Binns
MD, MA (Moral Sciences), FRCGP, DCH, DObstRCOG

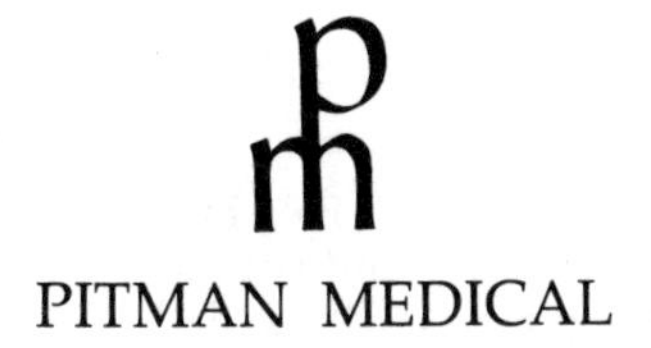

PITMAN MEDICAL

First published 1978

Catalogue Number 21 0826 81

Pitman Medical Publishing Co Ltd
PO Box 7, Tunbridge Wells,
Kent TN1 1XH, England

Associated Companies

UNITED KINGDOM
Pitman Publishing Ltd, London
Focal Press Ltd, London

CANADA
Copp Clark Ltd, Toronto

USA
Fearon Pitman Publishers Inc, California
Focal Press Inc, New York

AUSTRALIA
Pitman Publishing Pty Ltd, Carlton

NEW ZEALAND
Pitman Publishing NZ Ltd, Wellington

British Library Cataloguing in Publication Data
Elliott-Binns, Christopher
Medicine.
1. Medicine
I. Title
610 R130

ISBN 0-272-79511-9

Set in 10 on 12 and 9 on 10 VIP Palatino,
printed by offset-lithography and bound
in Great Britain at The Pitman Press, Bath

Contents

Acknowledgements

I wish to thank the following for their help in the preparation of this book: Drs Bernard Baillon, Kevin Fogarty, John Toby and the many other friends and colleagues, my partners in particular, with whom I have discussed these matters over the years; members of my own family for their wealth of knowledge and common sense; David Dickens for his guidance and wise counsel; the Editor of *Medical News* for permission to include several case histories previously published in the series "Consultation Point"; Dr John Fry and the Panel on Self Care for permission to include the diagram on page 91; Diana Butcher, librarian to the Cripps Postgraduate Centre, Northampton for her help with research; Mrs D. Barrington for typing the manuscript; and finally, if one is permitted to thank a building, St John's College, Cambridge for providing the tranquillity where this book was largely conceived and partly written.

Prologue

This book is about the Art of Medicine, which by tradition originated with Hippocrates, who has earned himself the title of the father of medicine. He was born and practised medicine on the island of Cos and by happy chance the letters COS stand for three important ingredients of the Art, namely Creativeness, Observation and Sensibility, and it might be as well to define these words straight away. Creativeness I take to mean imagination, originality, inventiveness. I prefer it to the term "creativity" which has become something of a technical expression, almost approaching jargon and, as the reader will soon find out, I do not like jargon. Observation, according to my dictionary, means – "accurate watching and noticing phenomena as they occur in nature". Sensibility is awareness, sensitiveness and tenderness towards people, objects and ideas. It is a good word because it suggests being sensible as well as sensitive.

This is not a book about the Science of Medicine, except in so far as art and science are intermingled. This does not mean that I am, in any way, opposed to the concept of medicine as a science. It is just that I happen not to be writing about it. Without science medicine becomes para-medicine just as without the practice of the Art it becomes a theoretical exercise. Nor does this book deal much with wider aspects of medical care, such as the organisation of health services and economic priorities which are rightly so much in vogue today. It is concerned, like Hippocrates, with illness, patients and doctors.

It is, therefore, a book with a built-in bias and the reader may find it helpful to read it in conjunction with some sociological work in which there is at least one graph or table on every second page, or with a textbook of medicine or surgery. Thus will his equilibrium be restored.

Some of my colleagues may raise their eyebrows because I have not, except in a few instances, given supportive evidence for my statements nor mentioned the names of writers whose work has a bearing in the matter under discussion. This is because, in my opinion, nothing disrupts the flow of a book so much as inclusions such as (Smith et al. 1972) or ($P > 0.01$). Footnotes are equally destructive. I must, therefore, excuse myself to my colleagues, to Smith et al. and to statisticians by merely saying "It is not that sort of book".

The main source of the book is the Hippocratic Collection. Excerpts from this work are identified by a reference number which indicates the volume and page of the Loeb Classical Edition (see Bibliography). This is important because the reader may wish to look up the original, especially as I have found it necessary to do some paraphrasing with which he is at liberty to disagree.

The book is written mainly from the viewpoint of a British family doctor, working in the rather atypical situation of a national health service. I will use traditional British phrases, such as general practitioner for generalist, house surgeon for intern, surgery for office and home visit for house visit.

However, Hippocrates wrote for all doctors and the similarities between branches of medicine and between countries where it is practised are greater than the differences. What goes for general practice goes for medicine at large, and what goes for the United Kingdom, goes for all countries. The Art is universal.

Those who have sailed round the Greek Islands will know the winds are notoriously changeable. It took Odysseus ten years to get back from Troy to his home in Ithaca because of these shifting winds and other more exciting hazards. In this book I will be blown off course sometimes by my shifting ideas but always I will come back to Cos.

1

The Art of Hippocrates

No-one reads Hippocrates nowadays, that is to say no-one apart from a few Greek scholars and some devotees of medical history. Choose a qualified doctor or medical student at random and ask him what he knows about Hippocrates. He will, of course, mention the Oath but will not remember much about it because the swearing of the Oath is no longer part of becoming a doctor. He will almost certainly quote, "Life is short. Art is long", but if you presumed to ask him what it meant he might well be unable to tell you. Hippocrates is, of course, the father of medicine but he appears to be dying from natural causes. Can we revive him? Has the Art he practised and wrote about been forgotten?

One cannot blame our randomly selected doctor for not having read Hippocrates because it must be said at once that much of the so-called Hippocratic Collection is unreadable, that is to say it is for the modern reader irrelevant, unintelligible or so obvious as to be tedious. This may sound a terrible condemnation of a man who is generally accepted to be a great writer but anyone who doubts it should set himself the task of reading the thousand or so pages. None the less the Collection contains the principles on which the Art of medicine was founded and on which, I contend, it still depends for its inspiration and guidance. The task I have set myself is to extract the essence, to write down the memorable passages that leap at the reader from the long-winded text, then to show that they are not only up-to-date but often ahead of our time. One does not look back to Hippocrates, one looks forward.

In doing this I am taking a liberty – and it is a liberty – because my knowledge of Greek is negligible so I cannot go to the source to seek what Hippocrates meant. I have to depend on translations. In the Loeb Classical Library, which can be found in any sizeable library, the Greek and English are set on adjacent pages. The translators, W. H. S. Jones and E. T. Withington, produced a four volume work of great accuracy and imagination. As they themselves admit, "imagination" is sometimes essential because many of the words are not to be found in a Greek dictionary. Also some of the passages are obscure, others nonsensical, so at times the authors have despaired and written a paraphrase as a footnote. Their mistake is, I believe, to have used an outmoded form of English. Because Hippocratic medicine resembles the art of medieval times more closely than present day science the translation abounds in such expressions as "coction", "ague", "flux", "alvine", "clysters" and other words not within the repertoire of today's medical student or doctor. Although the reader may enjoy this medieval aura for a few pages he will soon get bogged down because he is having to do a translation of a translation as he goes along. This is almost an impossibility, and he will rightly throw the book down in despair and turn to something more entertaining.

For this reason I have selected only a small number of worthwhile passages and have transcribed them into reasonably modern English. My great ally has been Roget's Thesaurus. For those who are not familiar with this fine book I must explain that it gives alternatives or finer shades of meaning for almost any word you can think of. I like to assume that I have come nearer to what Hippocrates really intended to say by this method rather than referring to a Greek dictionary. Also I like to think the quotations have become more relevant to present day thought. Some are unchanged from the original text, others are paraphrases because they have to be to make sense.

Let me give an example. One famous aphorism exhorts the

doctor not only to do his duty but "to secure the co-operation of the patient, of the attendants and of externals". I have changed this to "secure the co-operation of the patient, the staff and relatives". This is not exactly what Hippocrates said but it is, I think, how he would have put it had he been alive now. Words and ideas change and the truth is what is true for today.

Take as another example the word Holy. Hippocrates insisted that a doctor should keep his personal life holy, but the meaning of the word has changed so much that if nowadays you were to call someone holy he would take it as an insult, unless he happened to be a guru. Pure is a possible equivalent. A scientist knows what a pure metal is and a poet understands the purity of a mountain stream but this, too, has unfortunate connotations, suggesting lack of sexual drive – a good description of a maiden of unimpeachable character but not of a practising doctor who sees the world as it is in its degradation as well as beauty. These are what I call spoilt words, and a spoilt word is spoiled forever. If one searches for a more modern equivalent one might think of "dedicated", "moral" or even "well integrated" but these hold but a fraction of the original meaning of the word Holy.

I have taken another liberty. The worthwhile passages are scattered through four volumes and I have grouped them according to subject matter rather than their position in the text. In doing this I open myself to the criticism that I have selected passages at random, arranged them out of context and interpreted them as I thought fit. My defence is to concede the point. My excuse is that this is the only way that I, a practising family doctor, can make sense of the Hippocratic Collection. The conclusion is that this is a personal view of Hippocrates and the reader is asked to accept it as such. This book is for the general reader, not the scholar.

Who was Hippocrates? He was the professor of the medical school of Cos, a Greek island lying near the coast of the present day Turkey. The geography is important because it was in the towns of this coastline, called Ionia in those days, that the Greeks began to think scientifically. Hippocrates was probably born in 460 B.C. and no-one knows for certain when he died, but he is said to have lived to a great age. His life coincided with the incredible upsurge of human thought associated with Greece in general and Athens in particular. He was a contemporary of the philosopher Socrates, the dramatists Sophocles, Euripides and Aristophanes, the traveller Herodotus and the historian Thucydides. His life span overlapped those of Pericles, Pheidias, Aeschylus, Plato and many other names associated with Classical Greece. He lived through the anxious times of the Peloponnesian War when for thirty years Athens and Sparta did battle like the proverbial whale and elephant. It was thus paradoxically a world of decay as well as a world of progress. Ideals were conveniently put on one side in the exigencies of war.

He was not the founder of the medical school of Cos but he became its chief professor and father-figure. Tradition has it he dispensed his knowledge by holding interesting seminars under a plane tree. This tree is still to be seen today, rather decrepit and propped up with pieces of wood, which seems a remarkable feat of endurance for a plane tree whose normal span of life is 500 years. It is more likely to be a seedling from the original stock, carrying on the tradition of its ancestor by providing shade for scholars.

Hippocrates was probably the son of a doctor of the same name and his own sons were eminent physicians which suggests that the practice of medicine was very much a family affair in those days. He travelled widely and is said to have visited Athens during the plague which not only killed one third of the population but destroyed the optimism of a growing culture. History books show pictures of a bearded gentleman "thought to be Hippocrates" who looks very much like the other bearded gentlemen of his day.

No-one claims that Hippocrates himself wrote the entire Hippocratic Collection which consists of some seventy books or articles produced over a period of about two hundred years. One can only surmise that the collection is partly based on the ideas evolved during his professorship at Cos and formed the reference library of its medical school.

Hippocrates finds himself in a position similar to Homer because no-one knows if the Iliad and Odyssey were written by

Homer alone or if they are a collection of folk-lore based on history. Just as it is more rewarding to think of Homer as a poet rather than a board of editors, so it is more rewarding to think of Hippocrates as a doctor of great distinction and original thought rather than a reference library. Besides one cannot keep referring to any person as "they". Homer has the advantage of having written books which are a joy to read: this is only partly true of Hippocrates.

Hippocrates has made his mark on the history of the world for two reasons. First, he comes to us across the centuries as someone of enormous wisdom and integrity. Second, he introduced a new way of thought in medicine and science. To understand the second of these statements one must have some knowledge of the Greek way of thinking. At that time the Greeks, especially the Ionians, had a compulsion to *explain* everything. Because they had little of the basic knowledge we have today they had to rely on all-embracing concepts. In other words they used a philosophical approach. This does not mean they did not observe but their observations had to fit a pattern and for them the pattern was more important than the observations. If the pattern turned out to be wrong it was difficult to change and many of their errors became so ingrained as matters of faith that they were believed until very recent times. Fresh observations were used to support not to disprove their concepts, thus producing a curiously twisted idea of nature.

A well known example was the observation of the philosopher Empedocles that water can be present in various forms. It can be liquid (water), solid ice (earth), steam (air) or it can be sucked up by the sun and become fire. He therefore deduced that the physical nature of matter was earth, air, fire and water and these were interchangeable – a very reasonable deduction but, unfortunately, incorrect as a general concept.

Similarly a study of the secretions of the body suggested there were four essential elements or "humours" – phlegm, blood, yellow bile and black bile. This came to be regarded as the true nature of the body and formed a false basis for the study of medicine which was not finally discarded until the nineteenth century A.D. Yet in the age of Hippocrates the idea was reasonable and certainly more logical than magic or "acts of God". People no longer believed that Apollo, the archer-god, struck patients down with his fierce darts during a time of plague, although they clung to the idea that epilepsy was divine, that is to say beyond natural laws.

They were also slow to abandon the idea that illness was a punishment for wrongdoing and it is interesting that the Hippocratic Collection was written at about the same time as the book of Job. Readers of this superb dramatic poem will remember that Job suffered a series of disasters including a crop of boils but, after much discussion, it was decided this was in no way Job's fault. An unbiased reader would consider that Job was unfairly treated by a divine power who made amends by belatedly presenting him with substitute wives, children and cattle. God was all powerful and neither Job nor anyone else had a right to criticise him or bewail his own fate.

The heroes of Greek Mythology suffered in similar way from the whim of the gods, and anyone who reads Homer's Iliad will become disgusted by the casual way the gods treated mortal men who were only doing their best. We cannot lightly forgive the goddess Athene for tricking Hector into turning to fight Achilles, then depriving him of a spear at the critical moment. He had too much to contend with as it was.

However, the great dramatists of Hippocrates' time were introducing the idea that the fault lay in the people themselves rather than fate. Even if their downfall was predestined it was their own selfishness, pride and stupidity that led them to it. It can be claimed that Greek Drama was the beginning of modern psychology, leading on the one hand to Freud, on the other hand to Shakespeare.

Turning to physical illness, we must remember that Hippocrates was not in a position to understand disease in the same way that we do today. There was no acceptable method of classifying illness. The rival medical school at Cnidos attempted to do just this and caused disastrous confusion. Hippocrates writes disparagingly of them and the hostility between the two schools was intense. There is a story that Hippocrates, as a young man, crossed the water by boat and set fire to the Cnidian library. This is almost certainly apocryphal although medical students do get up to all sorts of tricks.

Hippocrates had almost no means of curing illness. Minor operations were sometimes successful and the knowledge of practical orthopaedics was quite remarkable. With these exceptions treatment was almost entirely symptomatic and not very helpful at that. Nursing and general care was all important, although this is assumed rather than described in the Collection.

What then could Hippocrates do? He could observe the illness without bias and by comparing it with other similar illnesses he could, to some extent, foretell the outcome. He called this Prognosis and much of his writing is concerned with this aspect of the medical art. Critics have said that he seemed to spend most of his time deciding when his patients were going to die then standing back to watch them do it. This is partly true but it omits to mention, as we have already said, that Hippocrates comes over as a figure of enormous sensibility. He did not stand back. He came forward and offered help and comfort. Much of his writing is about how a doctor can best do this and even his brief clinical "case histories" give an impression of compassion not callousness.

Part of his greatness was that he realised his own limitations and those of his art. No all-embracing theories could explain illness or lead to cure. It was only by careful study of the disease and the person suffering from it that a picture could gradually be built up. This study must include failures as well as successes and in 60% of his case histories the patient died. The later giants of medicine, like Galen, did not follow his example. Their patients always got better.

In short, Hippocrates was a scientist, one of the first scientists ever to have lived. He rejected a philosophical approach, although a true study of medicine must eventually lead to some kind of philosophy – not the other way round. In a similar way he rejected classification as an aid to observation, as practised by the Cnidian school, but realised that observation must eventually lead to a workable system of classification. This did not occur in his time nor for another two thousand years. People have criticised him for his nebulous attitude. The Cnidians at least tried. Or as W. H. Jones put it, "Hippocrates did the wrong thing well; the Cnidians did the right thing badly".

His ideas were new to his age and not readily understood. Some of the Hippocratic Collection is almost an exact contradiction of what has been said so far and it is tempting to believe that his followers were unable to escape from the net of philosophy. However, if we assume the Collection was a reference library, it is natural that some of the works did not belong to the true Hippocratic School. Even the wicked Cnidians may have slipped in a treatise or two. This is why much of the writing consists of tedious arguments based on false premises and is of no value today.

What was the purpose of "observation"? First, to learn the truth. Second, by learning the truth or even being able to give an accurate prognosis, the doctor understood the patient and the patient knew he was understood. It was partly a question of prestige, partly of human relationship. We can imagine that Hippocrates was not only an expert in bedside observation but also in the bedside manner in its best sense. This is why he laid so much stress on how a doctor should conduct himself in such matters as dress and speech.

He also saw the patient as part of his environment. The seasons, the weather, the local customs, were all important in understanding the disease and the patient. One of his most famous treatises "Airs, Waters and Places" was in use in medical schools and reprinted as recently as 1874. It is fortunate for us that Hippocrates was so interested in environment because it led him to write about politics and "culture" in general. His description of the ways of Barbarians is fascinating and sometimes amusing.

He stressed that the patient himself can influence his relationship to the environment by what is called Regimen. This, for the most part, was to do with diet and taking exercise. What better approach could there be when curative drugs did not exist or, the cynic might add, even when they do exist? Sometimes Hippocrates overstepped the mark and became a busy Mrs Beeton, devoting pages to the exact ingredients of gruel or broth for various illnesses.

I said at the beginning of this chapter that few doctors nowadays read Hippocrates. I suppose I am an exception because, for some reason, I bought his complete works when I first went into practice and marked the passages that interested me. The four volumes have stood on the mantelpiece of my consulting room ever since and sometimes I even take them down and look at them. This may appear a form of archaic amusement but in fact I believe strongly that all doctors should hitch their wagon to a star – provided, of course, they leave the knot fairly loosely tied. There are many other stars suitable for wagon-hitching, and I will mention some later, but for the present purposes Hippocrates is my star.

Those who consider this rather ostentatious should have at least a working rule of some sort. I have always admired the message Nelson sent to his fleet before the battle of Trafalgar: "In case signals cannot be seen or clearly understood, no captain can do wrong if he places his ship alongside that of an enemy". My working rule is: "In case signals cannot be seen or clearly understood, no doctor can do wrong if he does what Hippocrates would have done".

In the succeeding chapters I am going to record excerpts from Hippocrates' writings, comment on them and illustrate them with case histories from my own and others' experience. It is, therefore, fitting that I should start with some case histories written by Hippocrates himself. These are as he wrote them except that I have shortened them slightly. It may amuse the reader to try and come to a diagnosis, and the "answers" are given at the end of the chapter.

Case 1
(1.187)

Philiscus lived by the wall. He took to his bed on the first day with acute fever and sweating; night uncomfortable.

Second day. General exacerbation. Bowels open well with small enema. Restful night.

Third day. Fever subsided until midday. Towards evening acute fever with sweating, thirst, dry tongue, dark urine. A sleepless night, completely delirious.

Fourth day. All symptoms worse. Dark urine. A more comfortable night and urine a better colour.

Fifth day. About mid-day nose bleed with fresh blood. Urine varied with scattered round patches in it resembling semen, which did not settle. Suppository given with poor result and flatulence. A distressing night, snatches of sleep, irrational talk, extremities cold and would not get warm: dark urine, snatches of sleep towards dawn; speechless, cold sweat, extremities cyanosed.

Sixth day. About midday the patient died. His breathing throughout consisted of infrequent deep sighs as if he had to remember to breathe. The spleen was enlarged; cold sweats all the time. Exacerbations on alternate days.

Case 2 (1.203)

Crito, in Thasos, while walking about was seized with a violent pain in the great toe. He took to his bed the same day with shivering and nausea; regained a little warmth; at night was delirious.

Second day. Swelling of the whole foot which was red about the ankle and distended: black blisters: acute fever; mad delirium. He died on the second day.

Case 3 (1.233)

The youth who lay sick by the Liar's market was seized with a fever after unaccustomed fatigue, work and running.

First day. Disturbance of bowels with pale, liquid copious motions: urine thin and dark: no sleep: thirst.

Second day. General exacerbation: motions worse and more copious. No sleep: delirious: slight sweating.

Third day. Uncomfortable: thirst, nausea, restlessness, distress, delirium, extremities blue and cold, resistance but no swelling in both sides of the abdomen.

Fourth day. No sleep, worse.

Seventh day. Died. He was twenty years old.

Case 4 (1.267)

In Larisa a bald man suddenly experienced pain in his right thigh. No remedy did any good.

First day. Acute fever: the patient was quiet but the pain persisted.

Second day. The pain in the thigh subsided but the fever grew worse, the patient was rather uncomfortable and did not sleep: extremities cold: copious unpleasant urine passed.

Third day. The pain in the thigh ceased but there was delirium with distress and restlessness.

Fourth day. Death about midday.

Case 5 (1.277)

In Thasos a woman of gloomy temperament after a grief with a reason for it did not take to bed but lost sleep and appetite. She was thirsty and felt sick. She lived near the palace of Pylades on the plain.

First day. As night came she was frightened with much rambling, depression and slight feverishness. Early in the morning she had frequent convulsions and in between was delirious and uttered obscenities: pains all over, severe and continuous.

Second day. Same symptoms: no sleep: fever worse.

Third day. The convulsions ceased but were succeeded by drowsiness and heaviness of spirits, followed in turn by wakefulness. She would jump up: could not restrain herself: wandered a great deal: fever acute: on this night she had a heavy sweat and her fever dropped. She then slept and was perfectly rational. She had had a crisis. On the third day the urine was dark with particles which did not settle. Near the crisis copious vaginal bleeding.

Case 6

In Thasos the wife of Philinus gave birth to a daughter. The vaginal discharge was normal and the mother was doing well until the fourteenth day after delivery when she was seized with a fever accompanied by rigors. At first she suffered in the stomach and right hypochondrium. Pains in the genital organs. The discharge ceased. No sleep: extremities cold: thirst: urine thin and at first colourless.

Sixth day. Much delirium at night, followed by recovery of reason.

Eighth day. Rigor, acute fever: many painful convulsions: much delirium. No sleep.

Tenth day. Lucid intervals.

Eleventh day. Slept: complete recovery of her memory followed by quickly renewed delirium.

Fourteenth day. Much wandering with lucid intervals followed quickly by renewed delirium.

Seventeenth day. Became speechless.

Twentieth day. Death.

Suggested diagnoses –

Case 1 Malaria. Note the earliest reference to Cheyne-Stokes breathing.

Case 2 The first sentence suggests gout but the fulminating course rules this out. Could it have been a snake bite or scorpion sting? The Greeks wore sandals. Or perhaps septicaemia after treading on a thorn.

Case 3 Dysentery.

Case 4 Very difficult to diagnose. The suddeness and severity of the pain suggests an embolus or some other vascular disaster. With osteomyelitis the pain would have got worse as the fever rose.

Case 5 A fascinating history this. I suspect the gloomy lady's "grief with a reason" was an unwanted pregnancy. She induced an abortion which became infected. She was lucky to survive a severe septicaemia and complete her miscarriage. Her obscenities suggest she was a lady of ill repute.

Case 6 Presumably puerperal fever, in other words an infection of the uterus with septicaemia.

2

The Purpose and Meaning of the Art

1.17 *The art of medicine has come into being through necessity because an ill man cannot benefit by the way of life enjoyed by someone who is well.*

This is the first and foremost principle, often forgotten today. A doctor only succeeds if, as a result of his treatment, the patient enjoys life to a fuller extent that he would otherwise have done. This is not quite the same as the teaching in medical schools where a student learns to believe he is successful if he makes the right diagnosis. Usually they coincide but not always. The following case history is an illustration of this. It bring us with a jerk from the Greece of Hippocrates to the recent past in England.

Case 7 A young R.A.F. medical officer was posted to a head-quarters unit where he was condemned to carry out endless routine Annual Medical Examinations on offic-ers and aircrew, most of whom were extremely fit. One day while examining the abdomen of a senior officer he was able to feel the tip of the spleen. He referred the officer to a specialist and eagerly awaited the report. To his chagrin the specialist wrote somewhat abruptly that he was unable to feel the spleen but had arranged a routine blood test. A few days later the specialist 'phoned to say that the film had shown clear evidence of

> chronic lymphatic leukemia. He was gracious enough to congratulate the medical officer on his diagnostic skill and also wrote to his superior, commending his thoroughness. The medical officer was highly delighted. The patient was brought before a medical board and, although fully fit and active, was retired from the Service with a pension. He lived for many years without symptoms but found life pointless and disagreeable.

For the patient it was a disaster, for the medical officer a high spot in his career, for the R.A.F. the loss of an experienced officer. The moral is that the disease is only important if it is important for the patient. If it does not matter it is a luxury for the doctor. At that time there was no satisfactory treatment for leukemia and the patient's life was needlessly ruined. Yet the same story in less dramatic form occurs daily in hospital clinic or doctors' surgery.

2.193 *Medicine is this — to do away with the suffering of the sick, to lessen the disease, not to treat those cases where treatment is needless.*

What is meant by doing away with suffering? In Hippocrates' time it was an unattainable ideal since there were few beneficial medicines apart from opiates and alcohol, the pain relievers and tranquillisers of the day. Nowadays it is sometimes said that "no patient need suffer". As far as physical illness is concerned there is some truth in this remark, but not much. Many conditions cannot be controlled without reducing the patient to partial insensibility in order to obtain a pain free state, which is usually justifiable in terminal illness but not long term illness. If we consider mental illness it is even further from the truth. Relief of symptoms can be at the cost of alteration in personality, so in both cases it is a destructive process, although considered justifiable in some circumstances.

Until recently it was generally agreed that pain and suffering were a necessary part of life and it was as important to learn how to cope with them as to eliminate them. A woman must suffer travail before experiencing the joy of seeing her baby. An initiate to a tribe must suffer torture without wincing before becoming a man. The saint must experience the dark night of the soul before obtaining sublimity. Probably the distress was less because it was known to have a useful purpose and a foreseeable end.

Now this concept has largely gone by the board because of the doctor's power to do away with suffering. Why go through the Valley of the Shadow of Death when you can build a viaduct over it? Why suffer the pangs of childbirth if you can have an epidural block? Even going to the dentist has ceased to be an ordeal. The noise of the drill can soothe you to sleep.

Ivan Illich in his celebrated book on Medical Nemesis argues strongly against this medicalisation of life. The doctor's technique of relieving suffering is only one of many possible choices of coping with the problem, yet the patient is conned into believing he must follow this particular path.

Like all good prosecuting counsels Illich is careful to give one side of the case only. Chronic pain, however patiently borne, leads eventually to disintegration. Acute pain is less of a problem and can even bring satisfaction, which is, of course, retrospective. However, if it can be relieved most patients would wish this to be done, not only because of the immediate situation but because it frees them from fear of similar pain in the future. Clearly this is the doctor's task.

This is not to decry Christian Science or stoicism as a way of life. When the crunch comes, what patient with renal colic would refuse pethidine or what asthmatic would not want an injection in the early hours of the morning? Illich would agree with this if he had the misfortune to suffer severe distress, but his reminder is timely. Qualities such as patience, courage and endurance will never be obsolete, because no-one can escape suffering for ever.

2.203 *It is madness to demand from medicine a cure which it cannot give or for the body to resist a disease which is irresistible.*

Hippocrates was probably referring to infective illness, particularly the major epidemics such as the notorious plague of

Athens, where doctors found themselves useless. Nowadays we would think of old age which is itself irresistible. It can, however, be staved off for a time, often with no benefit to the patient or the relatives. Hippocrates would certainly not have countenanced euthanasia in any form but he would have had no truck with useless extension of life. To the Greeks and Romans death was commonplace, "a necessary end which comes when it will come", and it is only in recent decades that we have decided that death is wrong.

3.339 *Why trouble one's mind further about cases which have become incurable? This is far from the right attitude. The investigation of these matters belongs to the same science.*

This appears to be a contrary statement to the previous one but in fact it is not. Although a cure should not be attempted the doctor should remain interested in the patient and the disease because, as Hippocrates showed, the study of a fatal disease can be more academically rewarding than one that responds to treatment.

It is even more salutary now that post mortems are permitted, since in most cases they give a different answer from the clinical diagnosis. Hippocrates could at least pretend he was right. So could the top specialist of a hundred years ago. The present day specialist may be proved wrong at the final court of appeal, so he must retain some sense of humility. This is good for him and his patients.

1.299 *Whenever I enter a house I will enter to help the sick. . . . I will use treatment to help the sick to the best of my ability and judgement but never to do them harm.*

Nowadays it is more usual for the patient to enter the doctor's house, that is to say his hospital, clinic or surgery, rather than the other way round. This puts on the doctor the onus of being even more polite and considerate because he is the host rather than the guest. It also puts the patient at a disadvantage, especially if he has a long wait. The doctor should realise that a patient who has been sitting outside his consulting room for an hour or two, never knowing at what moment he will be called, can be reduced to a state of terror or apathy. Note that the doctor promises to help to the best of his ability and judgement. He does not promise to be right, and the "doing harm" implies *intentional* harm, otherwise no doctor could fulfil the Oath, of which this is a part.

1.313 *Time brings opportunity but for each opportunity there is little time. Healing is a matter of time but sometimes it is a matter of seizing opportunities. Knowing this a doctor must base his practice of medicine on experience and reasoning, not on plausible theories. A valid theory is a composite memory of things perceived by sense-perception which conveys to the intellect a clear image of the subject. The intellect, receiving these things over and over again, makes note of the occasions, the time and the manner and stores them as memories. Now I approve of theories if they are based on factual incidents and deductions from what is observed. But if they start as plausible fiction they create ideas that are worthless and obstructive.*

This passage requires elucidation. Time is often on the doctor's side because it leads to natural healing but none the less he must seize every opportunity and depend on his own repeated observation rather than theories which may or may not be correct. Unfortunately, although we pride ourselves that our theories are supported by factual evidence, they often turn out to be just as much "plausible fiction" as they were in the days of Hippocrates. It is an interesting exercise to study medical journals or textbooks of ten, twenty, thirty or forty years ago. It will be found that medicine is all too often an art of changing fashion although each fashion is made respectable by the scientific backing of the time.

A good example of this is the management of coronary thrombosis. Thirty years ago patients were kept in bed up to three weeks, lying flat and being shaved and fed by nurses. This was because it was shown that it takes an infarct three weeks to harden, so it was reasonable to assume that the heart muscle must have complete rest for this period. In fact prolonged bed rest increases the death rate and delays recovery. It may also produce a chronic invalid. Ten years ago anticoagulants were all the rage. Patients recently discharged from hospital queued up in droves for weekly blood tests, to their own detriment. It was tiresome and sometimes dangerous and meant they could not be let off the hook and lead normal lives. It is now accepted that anticoagulants are of little value in coronary thrombosis.

Yesterday's fashion was to pursue ruthlessly the cholesterol and lipids in the patient's blood stream. The outcome of these tests being rarely of practical value to the patient, attention has now switched to B-blocker drugs on a long term basis. These have good scientific backing but I would be unlikely to lose my money if I predicted they will be obsolete in ten years time. It could well be that patients by then will be spending three weeks in bed, with the luxury of being shaved by nurses. The wheel of medicine revolves and doctors and patients cling to it, trusting in the integrity of science with blind faith.

Many other examples could be given. Twenty-five years ago I worked for three months in a tuberculosis sanatorium during the winter. My time was spent walking through freezing wards or trudging from one snow-bound chalet to another. This was because fresh air was considered necessary for patients with consumption just as it had been in the days of Hippocrates. My chief practical task was to pump air into patients' abdomens to maintain a pneumoperitoneum. This was a hazardous job and has now been abandoned because it is known to be both useless and dangerous.

4.2 *A man's body consists of blood, phlegm, yellow bile and black bile. He enjoys the best health when these are balanced in activity, strength and quantity, in other words when they are equally mixed. Illness occurs when there is excess or deficiency of one element.*

I have included the theory of "humours" at this particular point because the reader cannot afford to laugh at Hippocrates' quaint ideas when we have just been discussing the only recently obsolete treatment of tuberculosis by insisting on having fresh air inside and outside the patient's abdomen. Even if the theory of humours is nonsensical the idea of health being a balance of opposites is very much up to date.

1.27 *Lack of certain substances causes harm and too much of them can do the same.*

It is one of the wonders of medical science that there has to be an exact balance between innumerable factors for the human body to work. A slight imbalance of a single chemical substance, enzyme or gene can be disastrous or even prevent the foetus from surviving. From tiny acorns great oaks grow and many serious illnesses are caused by apparently trivial faults. Cancer may be one of these.

The endocrine system is the most obvious example. Each gland is nicely in balance with itself and the other glands. It is often said that the pituitary gland is the conductor of the endocrine orchestra, but it is a very poor conductor because the instrumentalists tell it what to do. If the first violins think they are playing too fast they tell the conductor to slow his beat and he has no choice but to do so.

Health, for the thyroid, is a balance between thyrotoxicosis and myxoedema, for the pancreas a balance between diabetes and hypoglycaemia. The same Hippocratic principle can be applied to all parts of the body and the mind as well. The manic-depressive patient is healthy when his mania balances his depression. It has been said that the sane man is one who has every mental illness under the sun. If he lacks a particular mental illness he is in trouble. This is a little far-fetched but explains why a medical student or nurse who reads a psychiatric textbook will say "That's me!" at the end of each paragraph.

The following case fascinated me because it illustrated a Hippocratic balance between two different systems.

Case 8 Mrs S had the misfortune to lose her husband suddenly. She coped with her grief by throwing herself into various activities. She was skilled at toy making and worked hard at this to make ends meet and also to forget

> her sorrows. To the doctor she seemed anxious and overactive and he always spared time to let her talk about her problems and tried to induce her to have more rest. This he failed to do. After a year he was pleased to note she was becoming much more placid. Her words no longer tumbled over each other. However, she complained she was getting fat and once or twice mentioned she did not feel very well. The doctor paid little attention to this because he was delighted that her anxiety state was abating. However, when she started complaining of feeling cold and remarked she now sang alto instead of treble he decided to examine her ankle reflexes. He found the classical delayed reflex of hypothyroidism and tests confirmed the diagnosis of myxoedema.

The interesting feature was that the symptoms of anxiety and myxoedema balanced themselves out, giving an approximation of normality. Treatment of the myxoedema speeded up her toy making but she once more became anxious. Happily she has now attained a balance, being slightly hypothyroid and only a little anxious. She also feels well and admitted she had "been fighting against being slow". It had been a pseudo-normality and not true health.

1.43 *If the heat and cold of the body are equally mixed there is no illness because heat balances cold and cold balances heat.*

In other words the patient is euthyroid.

2.229 *Medicine is in fact subtraction and addition, subtraction of what is in excess and addition of what is lacking.*

The concept of balance of opposites applies to treatment as well as disease. Unfortunately nowadays the thing that is in excess may be the medicine itself, and Illich considers that there is a world wide epidemic of iatrogenic disease. "The Medical establishment has become a major threat to health." This again is something of an overstatement, but I sometimes shudder to think of the damage I have done in the past by giving large doses of digitalis to patients in heart failure. I am also sometimes pleasantly surprised to find how well some old people do when I take all their tablets away. However, even if one is a cynic, one must accept that modern therapy is enormously beneficial while remembering the corollary that any drug which is of value is also potentially lethal and will harm some patients. Often it is obvious when the treatment is creating the disease, but sometimes the connection is remote. The reader is asked to study the following case carefully. He can award himself full marks if he solves the problem.

Case 9

Mr H., a man of 48, visited the doctor because he had felt unwell for a week, with poor appetite, nausea and slight swelling of the ankles. He said he had not seen a doctor for years but had been attending a dentist for persistent toothache. On examination the doctor noted slight jaundice. The liver and spleen were not palpable, but there was moderate ankle oedema and also possible ascites. The last two factors suggested a more ominous diagnosis than infective hepatitis. A biochemical profile showed hepatic damage (bilirubin 4·6mgm, alkaline phosphatase 24 KA units, SGOT 450 units) and a low serum albumin, which explained the oedema. He was admitted to hospital where batteries of tests were carried out with no significant findings. He was treated with diuretics and injections of Vitamin K and the condition cleared up gradually, the liver function tests falling to normal. No diagnosis was made, so this is the point where the reader should demonstrate his intellect by careful thought.

A year later almost exactly the same thing happened, again following a bout of toothache. There seemed no possible relationship between jaundice and toothache but it turned out that on both occasions the patient had taken large quantities of paracetamol for the pain. The final diagnosis was paracetamol hypertoxicity. The doctors had forgotten about iatrogenesis, although in this case it was the patient who had created iatrogenic disease.

2.85 *A doctor's study should include consideration of what is beneficial to a patient's way of life while he is in good health.*

The base line a doctor must work from is the way of life and attitudes of the patient when he is well. One man may play squash or tennis several times a week, another may object to walking fifty yards from the car park to the office. A 'teenager may consider that going to bed at 3 a.m. is sensible behaviour while a middle-aged man may feel it necessary to go to bed each night after watching the ten o'clock news on television. Each person tends to find his own norm of behaviour and for him this is usually beneficial. Not always, of course, and the doctor may need to change the patient's life by gentle persuasion or reading the riot act. The important thing is that the doctor should have some idea what the norm is. If he does not have this vital information he cannot even decide if the patient is ill. Illness is a purely relative term and the decision may be the doctor's or the patient's or an act of collusion between the two. The benefits of illness may be vast, from avoiding the washing-up to being permanently off work. The disadvantages may be even more terrifying. Illness is, therefore, an important "diagnosis" in itself.

2.229 *Knowledge of cause of the disease enables one to administer what is most helpful.*

This may seem a statement of the obvious but it is often forgotten. Most doctors most of the time treat their patient's symptoms and have little time or intention of finding out the cause. It depends, of course, what one means by "cause", and according to the onion theory of illness there is always yet another cause behind the one the doctor is considering. He goes on peeling the onion forever and never reaches the centre even if he were to have the patient lying on a psychoanalyst's couch day after day for years, or hitched eternally to a computerised monitoring apparatus.

To take a simple example, a little boy is brought to the doctor because he has a cold. The cause is a virus. The doctor cannot remember which one and it doesn't matter anyway. The cause of the mother bringing the child is that he coughs at night and keeps his father awake, which makes the father irritable at breakfast next morning. The cause of her thinking it worthwhile bringing the child is her delusion that the doctor can cure the cold by prescribing an antibiotic. The cause of this delusion is that *her* mother used to take her to the doctor for antibiotics and series of doctors have accepted this as reasonable. Of course the real cause is that she is frightened of her husband's anger at breakfast especially because their sexual life is unsatisfactory and she is afraid of losing him to another woman. Her own father had deserted her mother when she was a child. And so on and so on. The centre of the onion is inaccessible. The doctor may be wise to peel off only one or two layers. At every consultation he must decide how much illness he will allow the patient, while the patient may decide how much illness he can insist on the doctor accepting. Often the easy way out is for the doctor to prescribe penicillin, which is the same as saying, "I admit your child is ill and let's leave it at that".

1.27 *It is hard to make one's knowledge so exact that there is little room for error. I would praise a doctor who makes only small mistakes. Precise truth is rarely found.*

Medicine is not an exact science and those who try to make it so will be disappointed. This applies not only to clinicians but also to those who work on the more technical side, such as biochemistry or even computerisation. Medicine implies judgement and the aim is to train oneself to make better and better judgements. It is, of course, undesirable to make many mistakes but equally undesirable to be afraid to make any mistakes at all, to the extent of taking no responsibility. The doctor who sends to hospital every child with abdominal pain, in case it might be appendicitis, is a menace. The doctor who is prepared to wait may occasionally delay admission but will find it rare for this to have any serious ill effect. Those who never make mistakes seldom do much positive good.

2.55 *Do not regret the omission from my account of the name of any disease.*

Because Hippocrates could not classify disease he saw each case as a "problem". In this age of the "problem-orientated approach" he would have been considered very modern in his attitude. The wheel has turned full circle, but will no doubt go on spinning.

2.65 *A mere variety of name is supposed to constitute a variety of illness.*

This is a deception found in textbooks and journals and practised on innocent medical students by their instructors. To give a disease a name is not the ultimate answer. Sometimes it implies a diagnosis, sometimes it does not. Often it is a form of defence for the doctor.

If a housewife comes to talk to a doctor about her problems he may write "Anxiety State" on her notes, but this is only a signpost not a destination. He could equally well write emotional problems, psychoneurosis, or domestic stress and be no further forward. He might even write "Anxiety State – Valium 2 mgm tds", which is a false or lazy diagnosis–plus–treatment.

In physical conditions the doctor must assess the precision of each name. Pernicious Anaemia is a clinical entity, Megaloblastic Anaemia a problem, and Anaemia a vague statement or even a guess if a blood test has not been carried out. Expressions like diarrhoea and gastroenteritis are used as alternatives, which is incorrect, since one is a description of a symptom, the other a claim, probably unverified, of the condition of the intestinal tract. It is only justifiable to differentiate illness when the names used are on the same level of precision. A surgeon who has carried out endoscopy can distinguish gastric ulcer, duodenal ulcer and hiatus hernia and make a statement accordingly. A family doctor can distinguish epigastric pain starting half an hour after meals from heartburn, but if he calls the second oesophageal reflux and the first peptic ulcer, he is doing no more than reminding himself of the likely cause. Careful attention to the meaning of words clarifies thought but few people nowadays are interested in words.

2.91 *In my opinion the aim of intelligence is to discover what was unknown before, provided the discovery is worthwhile, and this brings fulfilment to what was partly known.*

Note "provided the discovery is worthwhile". But there is a trap here. An ordinary medical reader may find articles in a journal which appear a complete waste of time, but he is not always in a position to judge their relevance. If a new form of haemoglobin is discovered in guinea pigs in Swaziland mankind may benefit in the long run. He probably won't, but he may.

Research that proves the obvious is hardly worthwhile. A paper I read many years ago showed that family doctors are usually busier on Mondays than other days of the week. I myself once carried out a bit of abortive research in which the only positive statistical result was to prove that grandmothers are usually older than mothers. If the result had worked out the other way round Einstein would have had to look to his laurels.

Another trap is to make a massed statistical assault on a collection of data. By the very nature of statistics erroneous results will crop up from time to time. A blind man shooting arrows in the air will eventually hit the centre of the target and to use statistics in this way is a form of blindness.

1.315 *Pronouncement and discussion are deceptive and treacherous. One must hold fast to facts even when making generalisations. One must stick to facts if one is to acquire that adaptable and accurate form of thinking we call "the art of medicine".*

Hippocrates hammers out this point again and again. If a doctor starts with things as they are he is at liberty to go on theorising, generalising or philosophising for as long as he has the inclination. He must, however, keep in mind the basic facts and if he does this he will soon know if he has strayed off the path or, as often happens, has gone in a loop and come back to it again. Medicine is a practical art, while "pronouncement and discussion are deceptive". After a stimulating and enjoyable discussion or case conference a doctor should ask himself two questions. In what way has this helped with the management of the patient or disease he has been talking about? In what way has this improved his skill as a doctor? Sadly, he will probably find the answer in both cases is "very little". This should not make him too despondent because his enjoyment has, in itself, been beneficial and the patients will profit from his renewed interest in medicine.

2.287 *A doctor should understand how he earns his income, be able to make friends and learn to live with his family and provide for them.*

This takes us off at a tangent. Until now we have been thinking of the Art of Medicine as an institution for the benefit of the patient. It is also a profession, that is to say a means of earning a living for the doctor, and Hippocrates was realistic enough to consider this. The extract above is strikingly modern and worth studying piecemeal.

A doctor should understand how he earns his income. He should realise that his practice is a business and run it on business lines. This is accepted as obvious in the U.S.A. and most countries. In Britain the National Health Service clouds the issue, especially for those doctors who work in hospitals and are largely salaried. Even so they should know how they earn their money, or at least employ an accountant who can explain it to them in a way they understand.

Hippocrates would agree that a doctor should ensure that he earns what he deserves. His profession comprises the factors which demand a high income, namely – hard work, a long training, great skill, a burden of responsibility and worry, a valuable service to mankind. Hippocrates would, however, be scandalised by the exploitation that sometimes occurs and would be bewildered by the idea of doctors going on strike or "withholding their services". He would sympathise with the concept that medicine is a vocation and money does not matter but would realise that this is impracticable for all except a few, but a very important few who are the white-hot core of medical idealism.

A doctor should be able to make friends and live with his family. This seems a strange statement but it is remarkably perceptive. Many doctors are so committed to their work and spend so much time with their patients that they become almost incapable of ordinary human relationships. Their professionalism is a shield, valuable yet dangerous, because it protects them from friends as well as enemies. To counteract this they must develop a life apart from their work, and their family is usually the chief source of natural friendship.

The doctor should provide for his family. Again an apparently obvious statement. A doctor may find it difficult to work enthusiastically if he knows he is not earning enough to give his family the way of life he thinks they should have. Unfortunately, in Britain today, this is a common situation, leading to bitterness and antagonism to the system. A little of this must reflect on the patient.

Just as important is the provision of a satisfactory relationship. A doctor must have time to be a husband or wife, father or mother, and if work prevents this it is essential to take stock. Many a doctor's family has fallen apart because the doctor has formed a habit of being busy even though his working hours are no more than those of other people. One elderly general practitioner told me that when his children had measles he did not hear about it until they were better. This refers to the bad old days. Now doctors, like chimney sweeps, are more humanely treated.

The art of medicine is concerned first and foremost with the patient's health and happiness, but the doctor's health and happiness is also important. The correlation between the two aspects is remarkably high. It is as unusual to have an unhappy doctor giving a patient a good service as a discontented patient giving a doctor satisfaction in his work.

Lay people usually assume that doctors must be happy because their work is so interesting and they have prestige and comparative wealth besides. This is based on the fallacy that because they are interested in their own symptoms the doctor will be too. Other fallacies are perpetrated by television serials and paperbacks, but contrary to general opinion, medicine is not all fun and excitement. An unusually perceptive patient said to me the other day, "I can't understand, doctor, how you can bear to sit and listen to peoples' troubles hour after hour". How indeed can I or any other doctor bear it? Other peoples' troubles are, in truth, essentially boring and the worst fate I can think of is having to listen to a maiden aunt talking about her aches and pains while the sun is shining outside or one's favourite programme is going to waste on T.V. Yet doctors spend much of the day doing this sort of thing.

This leads one to the conclusion that to be happy a doctor, or nurse for that matter, must *create* interest in his work. There are innumerable ways this can be done and each doctor has his own methods, which he varies from patient to patient.

The traditional method is to be interested in the disease. If the maiden aunt's aches and pains are just aches and pains, it is impossible to be attentive. If they are potential polymyalgia rheumatica, cranial arteritis or secondary neoplasia they are professionally stimulating.

The other common method is to be interested in the aunt. Why, anyway, is she a *maiden* aunt? What is the saga of her life? The turns of expression, the veiled hints, even the way she scratches her nose are fascinating studies in human behaviour.

If the worst comes to the worst the doctor may shut off and think about something else – a professional accomplishment which can give great pleasure. Or he may have devised a system of note taking which is so complex that he has to work hard to record what the patient is saying. All these are legitimate forms of behaviour to help the doctor overcome boredom in those cases where boredom is the chief obstacle.

This chapter has been about the purpose and meaning of the Art but we have, to a large extent, skirted round the subject. Hippocrates had the ability to go straight to the point. The following words should be engraved on the cerebral cortex of all doctors:

1.165 *Take a careful history of the past, diagnose the present state, try to foretell the future. As for the disease itself make it a principle to do two things – first to help and second to do no harm. In the art of medicine there are three factors – the disease, the patient and the doctor. The doctor is a servant of the art. The patient must co-operate in fighting the disease.*

3

The Patient, the Doctor and the Art

1.165 *. . . In the art of medicine there are three factors – the disease, the patient and the doctor.*

If one takes the "disease" first and thinks about it carefully one will come to the conclusion that there is no such thing. The word "pneumonia" for example is hypothetical. There are patients with pneumonia and there are lungs affected by pneumonia, but pneumonia itself is a fiction. In other words disease only exists in its relationship to the patient's body or mind and one may add that it only exists officially if given a name by a doctor. The disease, patient and doctor are inextricably woven together. Of course sometimes the patient does not wish his illness to become official and many ill people decry "sickness" and good luck to them. Others have personal reasons for not involving a doctor. A youth I saw the other day had been shamefacedly concealing the "clap" following "indulgence in venery and sexual excess", as Hippocrates would have put it. When he at last summoned up courage to come to the surgery he obviously received much needed help, physical and mental. As I wrote the word "gonorrhoea" on his notes it crossed my mind that the act of writing had created a disease because the third part of the triumvirate of patient, illness and doctor had at last been added. Some illnesses never reach this point:

> "Full many a flower is born to blush unseen,
> And waste its sweetness on the desert air."

Perhaps not a very apt quotation under the circumstances.

1.181 *I have made my judgements by learning from the nature of disease in general and from the particular nature of an individual disease: from the disease itself, the patient, the type of management and what sort of person the doctor is – for each has a bearing on the outcome, making it more or less favourable.*

Hippocrates rightly puts the disease first. The doctor is a doctor because he has studied the nature of disease. This makes him a different person from a social worker, priest or philanthropist, none of whom can do a doctor's job because they have not been trained for it. There is much confusion about this nowadays when doctors spend so much time dealing with emotional and social problems. The drift in this direction can go too far and a doctor should sometimes pause and consider what is his true objective. Is he doing work that could be done as well or better by someone else? It is a good idea to make a list of things which people would reasonably expect that only a doctor can do, such as physical examinations, operative surgery and diagnosis of complex illnesses. If he is doing practically none of these he should ask himself why he is there at all. An intelligent layman, with shrewdness and a little luck, could do as much and, let it be whispered in dark corners, laymen in the past have simulated doctors and done remarkably well. There are even cases on record of imposters being exposed and the patients signing petitions to retain their services. This is because they did part of the doctor's work very well, chanced the rest, and got away with it.

2.207 *Men with adequate knowledge of the art realise that some, but only a few, diseases have their seat where they can be seen:*

others, and they are many, have a seat where they cannot be perceived.

This is why the professional doctor will never be obsolete. Those who make superficial clinical judgements and give treatment without diagnosis do not have adequate knowledge of the art. Hippocrates showed great humility when he said few diseases are obvious. Today we like to think we hold the key to most illnesses. Even if we do it is the professional practitioner of medicine who knows how to use that key.

2.201 *The patient does not know what his illness is nor what causes it, neither does he know what to expect. He is given orders, suffering his illness at the time and afraid of the future: hoping for immediate relief rather than long term health: frightened of death but unable to endure his illness.*

Hippocrates shows his sensibility to the patient's feelings and at the same time summarises the motives in coming to the doctor. First he needs to know what is wrong with him and what to expect. Doctors often fail to perceive this and send the patient away with no explanation or, worse still, too complex an explanation. The following two cases show how easy it is for a doctor to fail in this respect.

Case 10 A housewife came to the surgery with the typical symptoms of cystitis. The doctor took a sample of urine, told her she had cystitis, and gave her a week's supply of ampicillin. Excellent treatment. Unfortunately she had no idea what cystitis was and for some reason got it into her head that it was a form of cancer. When the symptoms recurred a few days after she had finished the course of antibiotics, she was too frightened to come back to her doctor and hear the awful truth. She put up with three weeks' pain and anxiety, both of which were quite unnecessary and could have been prevented by thirty seconds of explanation of the meaning of the word cystitis and what she should expect.

Case 11 A man of sixty attended with a history of nocturnal heartburn. A young doctor told him he had a hiatus hernia and spent a long time explaining what it was and drawing diagrams on a piece of paper. The patient, who was of poor education, understood little of this but formed the impression his stomach had ruptured into his lungs. He called another doctor out at two o'clock the following morning because he was unable to breathe. A little reassurance put matters right.

The second reason for the patient's visit to the doctor is the obvious one, the relief of symptoms. A patient with severe gout, acute heart failure, or retention of urine does not want an explanation of what is wrong. He wants relief first, explanation second. The expression "I couldn't have cared less if I had died" is often used by patients after episodes of severe distress. Even if the symptom is a minor one most patients want relief, because that is what they have come for.

Case 12 A languid housewife attended the doctor with backache. He quickly spotted she had emotional problems – two naughty children, a husband who "went out with the boys" most evenings and an interfering mother-in-law. He spent a lot of time discussing this but as she got up to go she said in a plaintive voice, "But what about my back, doctor?" He should have given her advice or a prescription for aspirin before exploring her psyche. From a patient's point of view there is nothing more annoying than having a carefully cherished symptom casually cast aside by the doctor.

The third reason is the deeper one of fear of death which afflicts almost everyone over the age of forty, and many much younger. A cough may be the first sign of cancer of the lung, a stab of pain in the chest the precursor of a fatal heart attack, a slight irregularity in the periods the opening burst of gunfire in a long war of attrition ending in cachexia and death. Patients know this and something more than simple reassurance may be needed. It is what I call a sub-phobic state.

There are, of course, other reasons for the patient visiting the doctor which Hippocrates does not mention. Simple loneliness, a need to talk to someone. A certificate to be off work. Strange motives so deeply buried that the patient himself does not know what they are. An opportunity to dramatise himself. An excuse to come down town shopping. A form to be filled in. And so on.

1.17 *It is not easy for ordinary people to understand why they are ill or why they get better or worse, but if it is explained by someone else it can seem quite a simple matter. . . . If the doctor fails to make himself understood he may miss the truth of the illness.*

This stresses the two-way relationship. Not only does the patient get confused but the doctor misses the point and, sometimes, the diagnosis.

I have occasionally observed this when "sitting in" with a trainee doctor in general practice. Patient and doctor are at cross purposes. The doctor cannot make a diagnosis because he does not know why the patient has come to see him. The patient does not understand what the doctor is talking about because it is irrelevant. "Thank you anyway," he will say as he leaves the room, while the doctor has branded him as an "awkward patient".

1.325 *The doctor should exhort the patient not to worry about the outcome of his illness. He should accept responsibility so that the patient in his care will not get confused. If left to himself the patient, through the distress of his illness, may give up the struggle and die. But the doctor who takes the patient in hand and demonstrates his skill, preserving rather than altering nature, will sweep away the depression and anxiety of the moment.*

The patient is very much dependent on the doctor's professionalism. Kindness and sensible explanation may not be enough. The doctor should be seen to know what he is doing. If he is hesitant, changes his mind or even fiddles about with a syringe, the patient soon loses confidence.

Hippocrates' expression "preserving rather than altering nature" appears more applicable to his day than ours because nature was then the chief doctor. But it is still worth bearing in mind. Hippocrates' dictum was, "for the patient the least is best". Now, sadly, the attitude is often, "for the patient most is best". Nature is not given a chance.

One of my own patients returned from the Continent having suffered from what was obviously a mild traveller's diarrhoea, for which I would have given nothing apart from advice to drink plenty of fluids and avoid solids. She produced from a plastic bag five lots of tablets, three being antibiotics, which had cost her £33, and, incidentally, prolonged the diarrhoea. Treatment was stopped and nature performed a miraculous cure.

Horror stories like this prove nothing but suggest a lot. Conscientious family doctors in Britain fight a running battle with their patients not to prescribe antibiotics for illnesses which nature will cure. The doctor usually loses the battle.

Another way of interfering with nature is to admit patients to hospital, that is to say to remove them from their natural surroundings. Obviously this is often advisable and sometimes essential. Putting aside clinical reasons, the doctor has to decide if the patient would be happier and more at peace at home or in hospital. Hospitals can be noisy and frightening and there is a horrible tradition of waking patients at five o'clock in the morning, while in the evening the light is put out when they are at their most wakeful. Nurses are wonderful creatures but some patients are genuinely allergic to nursing. As Lord Melbourne said, "I would rather have men about me when ill than women; it requires very strong health to put up with women". That, of course, was before the days of male nurses. Hospital admission is a double-edged weapon and for many elderly people a death sentence.

2.313 *There is a close intimacy between patient and doctor and the patient puts himself in the doctor's hands. He must use self-control in relationship with women and girls.*

This intimacy is an extraordinary phenomenon which has been studied since medicine began. It is not "friendship", because a doctor cannot allow himself to be the patient's friend in the most precise meaning of the word. Indeed if he meets a patient on "friendly territory" it is often an embarrassment to both. A dinner party will be spoilt if the lady sitting next to him has, the day before, revealed to him her varicose veins or her psyche.

Similarly if he takes on a friend as a patient he is not doing them a good service because he will probably be singularly unsuccessful in making the transformation. The worst example of this is a doctor treating his own family. For one thing his treatment never seems to work. I have known doctors make the most ghastly and elementary mistakes in this situation. On the other hand a doctor's wife will often consider her husband callous and unsympathetic because he cannot play two roles at the same time. As a result the doctor's family, including the doctor, falls between two stools and is often deprived of adequate medical care.

If the patient is not a friend can one call him a client? This word, too, will not quite fit and one comes to the conclusion that a doctor–patient relationship is unique. There is an element of loyalty which is mutual. It is something like the Gurkha soldiers who used to say, "We do not mind if he is a good officer or a bad officer as long as he is *our* officer". The reader may think I am living in the past but this is the message I receive from Hippocrates, and, as I have said before, we do not go back to Hippocrates, we go forward.

Hippocrates himself probably did not analyse the doctor–patient relationship as writers such as Balint do today. (Balint's book "The doctor, his patient and the illness" takes its title direct from the Hippocratic Collection.) If he had done he would have used the family as a basis for the study of relationships because this was the Greek way of thinking. It is also something that everyone understands even if they pretend that the family is now out of fashion or is "an artificially induced transitory cultural phenomenon". If they believe this they are swimming against the tide as well as using unintelligible English. Readers of Desmond Morris's "Naked Ape" will know that close-knit family units were necessary for the survival of primitive predatory man and are still necessary for civilised predatory man.

At the time of Hippocrates the Greeks were learning about the complexities of human nature not so much through their philosophers and physician as through their dramatists, in particular the famous trio Aeschylus, Sophocles and Euripides. They wrote a lot about family feuds and family loyalties, in part symbolically, to the extent that some of their characters have become trade names for modern psychiatrists.

Case 13 Agamemnon was the not very efficient commander of the Greek expeditionary force against Troy. It is, however, fair to say that he had problems which General Eisenhower, in a similar situation, did not have to face. One of these was whether or not to sacrifice his daughter Iphigenia to the gods to allow the fleet to sail. He unwillingly decided he must do it, thus earning himself the hatred of his wife Clytemnestra and setting in train a course of events which became uncontrollable. In his absence Clytemnestra took a lover and on Agamemnon's return from Troy they murdered him in his bath. Another daughter, Electra, who had been excessively fond of her father, lived a sullen and rebellious life in her mother's palace. For seven years she brooded, and when her brother Orestes appeared on the scene the two of them murdered Clytemnestra and her lover in a brutal manner. In a last desperate attempt to save her life Clytemnestra bared her breasts to her son but this did not deter him from plunging the knife home. Electra was married off to a steady young man but Orestes, the matricide, was haunted by his guilt from country to country until he found refuge in Athens. Here he was put on trial and was found not guilty by the narrowest of margins due to extenuating circumstances.

This social worker's nightmare provided the themes for some of the greatest plays ever written and the foundation for a range of psychiatric symbolism. Similar themes abound in other myths and religions. To the Greeks the gods were a vast unhappy family, always quarrelling, intriguing and committing nasty deeds like rape and incest or, worse still, murder and cannibalism. But even through these traumatic incidents the family unit is apparent and that is why I think Hippocrates would have used it as a symbol of individual relationships.

Even today I believe the doctor unconsciously plays the family role suited to his own personality and the individual patient. If he chooses the wrong role there will be awkwardness and lack of communication. The role depends partly on the relative age of the doctor and patient, so if a patient requires a particular relationship he will choose a doctor of the right age, if he has the choice. It is difficult to make a newly qualified enthusiastic young man into a bearded sage and vice versa.

The most commonly accepted role is that of father. The doctor is spoken of as a father figure and Hippocrates himself is the father of medicine – although this has become a "spoilt" expression, individuals having been given the title of father to every art from car manufacture to pop music. None the less the reason that the doctor is a father is that the patients are often children.

This reversion to childhood is strange. The iller the patient is the more childlike he becomes. When a hardened industrialist is admitted to hospital for an operation he is treated like a child of six during the period just prior to the operation and for a short time afterwards. His stretcher becomes a cot and nurses call him "dear" and hold his hand. This is very necessary for him because he is completely subservient to his father the surgeon, and the nurses and other staff are his kin. He has to be told he's a good boy and be petted. Once he has recovered he may resent this relationship and I have heard patients complaining because the nurses call them "dear". "Sir" or "Mr Jones" is more suitable to their dignity. In the hospital clinic or family doctor's consulting room the situation is less extreme. I find I use expressions like "Let's have a look at your tummy, then" and I say "Bye, bye" when the patient leaves. This is not the sort of speech I would use in ordinary social relationships.

The second most likely role is that of an elder brother. The relationship is one of equality but the patient defers to the doctor's advice (we are talking of elder brothers as they used to be: nowadays they would be cheeked). This role is becoming more and more common and younger doctors I have spoken to consider it more usual than the father role. This is partly because the role suits their age-group better and partly because patients are becoming more adult in medical matters. Teenagers often resent any parental type of relationship with their doctor but cannot quite feel respect for a brother, so finally elect to have a distant uncle who is hardly in the family at all.

A third and very interesting role for the doctor is that of a husband. Ideally he should be the same age or somewhat older than the patient but this is not essential. It is especially likely to occur if the patient's own husband has failed her in some way, or if there is no husband because of death or separation. A doctor should not be afraid of this relationship which has little of the sexual in it and is mutually rewarding. It is, anyway, a part he should play well. It is probably most important in the event of widowhood, and many doctors have given support to a grieving patient of a kind a husband would normally give and helped the widow through to stability and possibly remarriage.

1.301 *I will abstain from all intentional wrong-doing and harm and will not abuse the privilege of examining the bodies of men or women, rich or poor.*

Of course the danger of the husband relationship, as people will gleefully point out, is that it can slide into a sexual relationship to the delight of Sunday newspaper readers. This happens extremely rarely due to a built-in check system with which every doctor is equipped.

It is extraordinary that a doctor can walk into a house, go upstairs and examine a woman naked in bed without even having to ask permission. Alternatively she will come to his consulting room and he will ask her to take off her clothes which she will do without reservation. There is no embarrassment in the naked or nearly naked body, but the act of undressing is not accepted and this is done behind a screen, or if there is no screen the doctor averts his eyes. To do otherwise would make him a Peeping Tom.

This extraordinary mutual understanding is almost foolproof and comparable with the many anti-sex systems used by animals. Richard Gordon describes an incident in one of his books, when the young ship's doctor is inveigled into entering a brothel in a South American port. When the hostess talks about her tummy pains, suggesting to him a diagnosis of gallstone colic, his sexual instincts are immediately switched off.

Case 14 The doctor was examining a patient in his consulting room at home when there was a power breakdown and the lights went out. He was forced to continue his consultation in candlelight. He found himself in the situation of pulling back the curtain, holding a three-stemmed candelabra above his head, and being confronted by the almost naked body of an attractive girl lying on a couch in flickering candlelight. The setting was so suggestive that patient and doctor were suddenly overcome by embarrassment. Fortunately a sense of humour prevailed. They both burst into laughter and shared the joke for a long time afterwards.

Although Hippocrates stressed that sex must be restrained, it happens from time to time that a doctor falls a little in love with a patient and the patient with her doctor. This can be beneficial provided it is kept within strict limits by both or confined to a world of fantasy. The very expression "falling in love" implies a good relationship even if it is socially inconvenient. Balint has described the doctor as a drug and sex is one of the components of this drug. The dose, however, is crucial and if this is exceeded the results can be disastrous, the complications of over-dosage being well-known. The best protection for the doctor is to be happily married.

I have assumed throughout that the doctor is of the male sex because it is awkward to write "he or she" in every other sentence. I am not in a position to describe the role of women doctors who, of course, may play the part of wife, mother or daughter. I have been told, however, that playing the role of wife is more complicated than that of a husband because wives are traditionally subservient, which does not fit in with the necessary dominance of the doctor over the patient. This can be a problem for women doctors.

What I have written is not unlike a homely version of Berne's "transactional analysis". He described human relationship as a presentation of one of three types of Ego – Parent, Adult and Child. The egos involved must interlock and with a doctor and patient it is usually a parent/child or adult-to-adult relationship. The doctor can rarely use his child ego professionally and if this element is strong in him he may find himself in difficulties unless there is some outlet away from his work. A young doctor may feel ill at ease with a patient of the same age and class as his own father because he has to suppress his child ego which would be inappropriate. The use of the word Ego is, I think, not very helpful because it implies a differentiation from a more basic Id, and this distinction is a product of the mind of the observer rather than the observed. However it helps to clarify what I have written, and transactional analysis is, in my opinion, a big step forward from traditional psychoanalysis because it is concerned with relationships rather than individuals.

I may have appeared to suggest that there should always be a close intimacy between doctor and patient. This, of course, is not so. If the reason for the visit is trivial or formal, which as often as not it is, the relationship may be of the slightest. Also a doctor at his busiest may purposely avoid intimacy, using a prescription pad or a throat torch as an intermediary. The personality or mood of either patient or doctor may be a bar to intimacy and most doctors have had the experience of being so mentally exhausted that they cannot have genuine contact with the patient and have to rely on their acting skill.

In my consulting room the patient's chair is purposely placed at the corner of the desk. A patient who wishes close personal contact will unconsciously pull the chair forward to be near to the doctor. The patient who wishes to have a barrier pulls the chair behind the desk when he sits down. This is a form of non-verbal signal. It may be added that the doctor on seeing who is the next patient on the list sometimes places the chair firmly behind the desk.

So we come again to the disease, the patient and the doctor. Between them they decide how close the relationship will be. "Human kind cannot bear very much reality" and both doctors and patients cannot always bear intimacy. This does not necessarily make them bad doctors or bad patients but they are not likely to be very good ones.

2.297 *Do your work calmly and efficiently but do not reveal too much to the patient. Give encouragement to the patient to allow himself to be treated: sometimes reprove him sharply and decisively and sometimes comfort him with kindness and attention.*

In spite of what has been said of family relationships the doctor should always keep himself a little aloof. He should preserve the balance between being dispassionate and being involved. Cases 10 and 11 showed how a doctor can say too little or too much. In the past doctors were expected to be tight lipped. This was part of their mystique, but to tell the truth they had few worthwhile secrets to hide and Hippocrates was modest enough to realise this. Now there are plenty of secrets but the patients, supported by the enthusiastic media, nose them out and consider it their right to do so. The doctor is, therefore, to some extent on trial and, as anyone who has appeared in court will know, it is better to say little and think carefully before you speak. Let the others do the talking.

This is a good principle in the consulting room or hospital provided the patient is not looked upon as "the enemy". The really expert doctor gets the patient talking and says little himself. He guides the patient to the right degree of understanding and merely adds the final coat of varnish. This is a counsel of perfection because some patients are so lacking in perception that everything has to be spelt out to them. Others benefit by being spoken to sharply and decisively, as Hippocrates says. This is best done as a matter of policy rather than in a fit of pique or rage, but even anger is an ingredient of the "drug doctor" and can impress the patient no end. Nagging never does any good.

Case 15 A doctor had for years put up with a middle-aged female patient coming to his consulting room to describe in tedious detail a vast panorama of symptoms. One day he flew into a rage and called her "a stupid selfish

> woman". She retaliated by calling him a "stuffed dummy". Since both observations were true the air was cleared and their relationship improved from that moment. The trouble had been that the doctor had felt and shown no interest in the patient and she had been compelled to elaborate her symptoms to impress him. It was a vicious circle.

This was an exceptional case and a doctor who loses his temper usually regrets it later because it has harmed him as much as the patient. On reflection he may realise it was not the patient's fault anyway. Very often an accumulation of minor annoyances build up to an explosion and I find myself that if I get cross about a patient I often take it out on the next-but-one patient on the list if he gives me the opportunity. This is unfair. It is also cowardly to be cross or sarcastic over the 'phone, because the doctor can be unkind without looking the patient in the face. He is also breaking his Hippocratic Oath because speaking on the telephone is technically entering the patient's house.

So we have this strange relationship between patient and doctor. Usually it is a simple matter based on common sense and politeness and with the aim of diagnosing and treating an illness. Too much should not be read into it. I have chosen family relationships as a model because they are easy to understand and I believe them to be the basis of Hippocrates' "bedside manner". I think it is wise to avoid psychiatric terms unless the situation is overtly psychiatric, which it rarely is. We get back to the onion again. How many layers should one peel off when examining the doctor–patient relationship? The answer is in most cases "None" because it is usually better to be unaware of the relationship. A mother reacts naturally to her child and may be confused by books on child care. In the same way a doctor usually reacts naturally to a patient and to study this relationship is to damage it. If he consciously decides to play the part of a father or husband he will probably find the consultation strained because the patient may not understand she is meant to be a daughter or wife and there will be a lot of confusion and ham-acting.

So the reader need not take too much to heart what has been

said in this chapter but study instead the following words written by Hippocrates which say it all.

2.287 *Medicine has impartiality, propriety, modesty, reserve in dress, logical thinking, good judgement, quiet forcefulness of character, purity, ability to express wide issues, knowledge of what is good and necessary in life, natural ability to help people, freedom from superstition, general excellence.*

The opposite qualities are intemperance, vulgarity, greed, lust, dishonesty, shamelessness.

4

The Practice of the Art

The Hippocratic Collection is in the main a manual of practical medicine, a textbook. The longest parts are about the practice of orthopaedics and the surgery of trauma. The Greeks knew a lot about fractures and war injuries. After all they were a warlike people and, centuries before, Homer had described with relish the exact injuries sustained by his heroes on the windy plains of Troy.

Case 16

When the mighty Achilles fought the Trojan warrior Deucalion he "pierced his forearm with the bronze point of his spear just where the sinews of the elbow are attached. Deucalion, waiting for him with his arm weighed down by his spear, looked Death in the face. Achilles struck the man's neck with his sword and sent head and helmet flying off together. The marrow welled up from the vertebrae and the corpse lay stretched on the ground."

Fractures were something which could be treated successfully even before the advent of plaster of Paris, and because the patient, if he recovered, had a normal life expectancy, the straightness or otherwise of the limb was a perpetual memorial to the skill of the doctor. One of the problems, then, as it is now, was extension of the limb when there was shortening and overlap and complicated racks and gadgets were devised to overcome this. Hippocrates would have saved himself a deal of trouble if he had invented Thomas's splint before Thomas did.

The following passage is included for the benefit of surgeons to show how little the basic principles of surgical technique have changed over 2,400 years.

3.59 *Requisites for the operating theatre; the patient, the surgeon, assistants, instruments, the light — where and how placed, their number, which he uses, how and when; the patient's body and the apparatus; the time, place and method. The surgeon, whether seated or standing, should be placed in a convenient position, the light shining on the part to be operated on.*

An admirably brief statement! And here is a description of the care of the hands.

3.363 *The nails should be neither shorter nor longer than the finger tips. Practise using the tips of the fingers, especially with the forefinger opposed to the thumb. . . . Practise all operations with either hand or both together, your object being to obtain skill, gracefulness, speed, painlessness, elegance and anticipation.*

2.227 *Habitual use is the best trainer of the hands.*

Much of the appeal of Hippocrates lies in his relevance. This passage could have come from a modern text book except that it would probably not have been so clearly written. Hippocrates was not by trade a surgeon. Doctors of his time were very much "generalists" and Hippocrates himself falls somewhere between a family doctor and a specialist, since he visited patients at home but also travelled far and wide as a consultant.

2.295 *When you enter a sick room you should anticipate what you must do before going in and have everything organised. For many cases need practised help, not reasoning.*

Organisation is important because it saves time and gives the patient a better service. It is of little value in itself although it is one of the legitimate ways in which a doctor may gain satisfaction from his work. Hippocrates is describing personal organisation, which is largely a question of anticipation.

For a family doctor not to have morphine in his bag when he visits a patient with severe coronary thrombosis is a more serious error than failing to hear a heart murmur with his stethoscope. Even getting an address mixed up or not having a coin for the telephone call box can be a disaster.

The hospital doctor who reads this may be smiling smugly but I have seen extraordinary errors in highly organised surgical units. After all, when a patient dies following a mismatched blood transfusion it can usually be traced to minor but preventable factors, due in turn to someone being tired or in a bad temper.

2.9 *For the more time you spend planning to meet an emergency the greater will be your power to save those who have a chance of recovery.*

A wise doctor will overhaul his routine frequently and even spend time *imagining* unforeseen disasters which may never occur, although most disasters do seem to occur once in a doctor's life time. It is also useful to do personal time-motion studies, not so much for emergencies as for everyday activities. It should, for example, be possible to syringe wax from a patient's ear or take a sample of blood in under two minutes if the necessary equipment is all within reach. It can, on the other hand, take ten minutes, during which time the doctor has walked thirty yards and possibly spattered his shirt with water or blood. A good routine allows the doctor to do whatever it is without thinking, which means he can talk to the patient at the same time.

There are many irritations in a doctor's life and these should be identified and, where possible, eliminated. This applies to such trivial matters as having prescription pads and forms within easy reach, but equally to snags which occur in major operative surgery. There are stories of surgeons becoming almost maniacal over trifling incidents such as not having exactly the right instrument available when a similar one would do equally well. I was told of an occasion when a surgeon whose brow was sweating asked a junior nurse to "mop". She promptly went out of the room, came back with a mop and started mopping the floor. He became so enraged that his assistant had to complete the operation. In retrospect this was amusing but at the time it was not and could have been prevented by simple instructions to the nurse about her elementary duties in the theatre.

Personal studies are valuable but I have little faith in large scale time-motion studies, which somehow seem to miss the point and attain nothing or even make matters worse. An attempt to rationalise an outpatient appointment system by distributing appointments more evenly during the morning led to the doctors sitting about doing very little for the first two hours, then rushing their work to get finished by lunch. The person who finds the answer to the outpatient waiting problem will rank with Pasteur and Banting and Best in the prevention of human suffering.

2.291 *The most convenient doctor's bag is one methodically arranged because the doctor cannot go through everything.*

It seems that doctors have always carried bags and even in Hammurabi's Babylon of 2000 B.C. the physician–priests carried little cases, presumably for incense and surgical instruments. The latter were used for cutting open sacrificial animals to study the state of the liver rather than for surgery on patients. This was much safer for both the patient and doctor because there was a law that if the patient died following an operation the surgeon had his right hand amputated. This was the ultimate in Medical Audit.

The commonly used bag today is the executive-type case with a foam rubber interior which can be cut to fit the shape of various instruments and bottles which are at once on view when the doctor opens his case. This is preferable to the miniature chest-of-drawers bag and vastly superior to the Gladstone bag, where the doctor was like a terrier at a rabbit hole in his frantic search to find what he was looking for.

I have heard people say it is an anachronism to carry a bag nowadays and the patient feels more at ease if the doctor arrives with a stethoscope and prescription pad concealed about his person. This is nonsense. The doctor's bag is an extension of the doctor and if he leaves it in his car he is unlikely to go back for a sphygmomanometer or syringe if these are needed. Not to have an adequate bag is bad clinical practice. A methodically arranged bag will make him almost as well equipped in the home as in the surgery.

2.295 *Make frequent visits; be especially careful in your examinations.*

A counsel of perfection of course but equally applicable to the consulting room or clinic as to the home. Diagnosis is often a product of time and repeated short consultations may be the best way of finding out what is wrong with the patient. A doctor who orders an urgent intravenous pyelogram will feel foolish when the radiologist diagnoses shingles because the herpes spots have appeared overnight. This, of course, is an extreme example, but with each patient a decision must be made. Does the doctor wait and see or does he launch at once into investigations? This is where experience tells and a young doctor may waste time and money because he does not use time as an ally. Many conditions, such as measles, are self revealing.

The second part of the quotation is, in a sense, the converse of the first part. Examination should always be careful but this does not necessarily imply a complete head to toe examination. Often a junior doctor fails because he has to be too thorough and so misses the obvious. He cannot see the wood for the trees, or rather an individual tree for the wood.

On the other hand a good initial examination may allow the doctor to decide with confidence that he need not see the patient again. It also protects him from legal difficulties if the unexpected happens.

2.65 *The whole of medicine should be studied. Everything that is good or right should be performed well and correctly. If it ought to be done quickly it should be done quickly; if neatly, neatly; if painlessly, with the minimum of pain; one should aim at excellence and doing things better than one's colleagues.*

"Quickly and neatly" are the key words for most patients, especially in general practice, "slowly and thoroughly" for the few. It is worth pausing to consider how a doctor can be both quick and efficient. The golden rule is not to appear in a hurry. An experienced doctor can complete a consultation in five minutes but give his patient the impression he has had all the time in the world. This is a knack. The young doctor has to unlearn the laborious system of the medical schools, the hallowed sequence of history, examination, diagnosis and treatment, or SOAP as the modern doctor may call it. SOAP means subjective, objective, analysis, plan, a new invention which means virtually the same with an added suggestion of hygiene, except that analysis is a better term than diagnosis.

With each patient and each disease a particular aspect of the procedure is paramount. When a patient says he has a bad back the doctor's first response could be "Let's have a look at it then". The history is taken while the patient is undressing and being examined, which does not take long with present-day clothing. (A colleague of mine declares that general practice came into its own when braces and corsets went out of fashion). This leaves time for the important part of the consultation, namely discussion about Regimen, as Hippocrates would call it. In backache, as in many other conditions, the way of life is usually more important than the diagnosis. The rarities such as ankylosing spondylitis, spinal secondaries or pain referred from other organs will be revealed by the doctor's clinical discernment or by his great ally, time. Although delay is undesirable it is not usually harmful.

In psychiatric conditions the history is supreme; in valvular disease of the heart, examination; in acute asthma, treatment. Each has its own importance and demands its share of the time available, so the doctor should be adaptable in his approach. Eventually he develops flair, or clinical acumen as it is sometimes called, and can jettison many of the disciplines of his training. He must, however, retain enough to prevent himself becoming slovenly in his work.

Excellence is the aim and to excell means to surpass. This by definition implies competition, so each doctor or unit should strive to become better than the next. More will be said of this later.

2.9 *First he must examine the face of the patient to see whether it is like the face of healthy people and especially whether it is like its usual self.*

However quick and neat the doctor is he must never fail to look at the patient, and it is extraordinary how often this simplest of examinations is forgotten. An observant doctor will often make a diagnosis before the patient sits down, especially if he knows the patient quite well. An unobservant doctor will be looking at his desk or prescription pad, which will teach him nothing. In a small survey I did for my own amusement I found I could make a good approximate diagnosis in 30% of patients before there was any exchange of words. The commonest and most obvious was "child with a cold and anxious mother". Other diagnoses often made were depression, anxiety, sciatica, sexual worries and bronchitis. Less common but obvious examples are anaemia, myxoedema, thyrotoxicosis, Parkinsonism, Bell's palsy and jaundice. I know of one case of severe jaundice which was missed in this way and another of severe anaemia due to a slow bleeding ectopic pregnancy, although the latter was admittedly seen in poor light. The patient, however, said, "The doctor never looked at me although he did put a hand on my tummy". A visual or snap diagnosis must, of course, be confirmed by the usual methods.

Quite apart from diagnosis, the initial glance is important because the doctor can, consciously or unconsciously, decide on the role he will play as described in the last chapter. Also he may choose the wrong opening remark if he has not looked at the patient's face. Two common examples are:

Doctor: Well, what's the matter?
Patient: (haughtily) That's for you to find out.

Or Doctor: What are you complaining of?
Patient: (in complaining voice) I'm not complaining.

The phraseology of the doctor's initial remark is important; he should have a repertoire from which he can select the right one.

2.9 *Nose sharp, eyes hollow, temples sunken, ears cold and contracted with their lobes turned outwards, the skin of the face hard, tense and parched, the colour of the face yellowish or dark.*

This is the well known Hippocratic Facies. In his day it signified impending death, an important diagnosis because the patient would wish to know if he was dying so that he could prepare himself. Today it signifies the urgent need for intravenous fluids and other methods of resuscitation. The diagnosis of impending death is now less important because it is usually presumed the patient will not want to know.

2.215 *When information is not available and Nature herself will yield nothing of her own accord medicine has found means of compulsion whereby Nature is constrained to give up her secrets without being harmed.*

If Hippocrates were alive today he would be amazed at the "means of compulsion" available. This would include blood tests, X-rays, examinations such as sigmoidoscopy, cardiac catheterisation and diagnostic laparotomy. The last two are sometimes referred to as "invasive techniques" or "insults to the patient", and Hippocrates was correct in saying there is a price to be paid for every secret nature is compelled to disclose.

The price must always be balanced against the likely benefits, whether it be frightening a child with the prick of a needle or undertaking dangerous investigations for a congenital heart lesion. Is it worth it from the patient's point of view? Is it worth it from the doctor's point of view? Is it worth it from the economic point of view?

2.211 *What escapes the eyesight is mastered by the eye of the mind. If the attendant cannot see the trouble with his eyes or learn it with his ears he tries to track it by reasoning.*

A doctor can become lazy and allow his reasoning powers to atrophy. A particular situation calls for a particular response and in hospital outpatients a doctor can order "the usual investigations" with a good chance of catching the diagnosis in the net. Similarly in general practice a doctor can reach for his prescription pad without thinking at all, in other words using a therapeutic net. This has some advantages because if a doctor is in bad form – maybe unwell or tired – he can switch to his "automatic pilot" and probably avoid serious mistakes, even if the patient does not benefit greatly from the interview. The Art of Medicine is, however, a reasoning art and the case below is an example of one which can be solved by reasoning alone. There is, I think, only one possible explanation for an unusual medical history and the reader is challenged to make the diagnosis on what he reads.

Case 17 The doctor received a call at 5.30 a.m. to see a patient of 60 who had woken with severe pain in *both* shoulders. This seemed a strange history. When the doctor reached the house he was met by an agitated daughter who said her mother had suddenly collapsed and she thought she was dying. The doctor hurried up the stairs expecting the worst. The patient was in fact fully conscious and did not look ill. According to the daughter she had suddenly "gone funny" and started breathing heavily.

On examination both arms were held to her side and the patient was unable to move either shoulder because of pain in the joint. It was noted there was a plaster cast on the left wrist and the doctor was told the patient had fallen down in the garden six weeks previously, knocked herself unconscious and fractured her wrist. The skull X-ray had been normal. At this point the reader is asked to consider the evidence and come to a conclusion, making the assumption that all the incidents described stem from a single cause, which of course is not always the case.

There are three occurrences to be explained:

1. A fall in the garden with loss of consciousness and a fractured wrist six weeks previously.
2. Both shoulders immobile and painful on waking in the morning.
3. A syncopal attack of short duration a little later.

The answer is Epilepsy.

1. The loss of consciousness was due to a fit, not a head injury.
2. An attack of nocturnal epilepsy caused bilateral dislocation of the shoulders. The patient was not to know she had had a fit in her sleep so woke up with painful shoulders.
3. A straightforward epileptic attack.

The doctor was helped to this diagnosis, which proved to be correct, because twenty years previously another daughter had had an eclamptic fit soon after childbirth and had dislocated both shoulders. The family was obviously "loose shouldered". Dislocation of the shoulders is a rare complication of epilepsy and is presumably due to arching of the back. It is difficult to think of other causes of severe bilateral shoulder pain present on waking although, before examining the patient, the doctor has in mind such conditions as coronary thrombosis and dissecting aneurysm.

In contrast the next case was one where nature gave up her secret by compulsion, with little productive reasoning by the doctor.

Case 18 A man of 32 attended hospital outpatients with a history of being thirsty and passing a lot of urine. He had also felt tired and irritable but had managed his work as an electrician in spite of the inconvenience of having to use the toilet frequently. Examination was normal and a routine urine test showed no albumin or sugar. The specific gravity was low (1006). A diagnosis of diabetes insipidus obviously sprang to mind, although the specific gravity was not as low as one would expect. The blood urea was normal. The doctor thought however the most likely diagnosis was hysterical polydipsia because the patient had personal problems which could well have produced these symptoms.

Fortunately, a second glance at the biochemical profile showed a raised calcium level (18 mgm per 100 ml). This led the doctor to look up polyuria in his textbook and he found hypercalcaemia listed as a cause. The patient was eventually cured by excision of a parathyroid tumour, with no credit to the reasoning power of the doctor who first saw him.

2.227 *The diagnosis of obscure illness is more a matter of opinion than factual knowledge, so there is the greatest possible difference between experience and inexperience.*

This is as true today as it was then. An experienced hospital consultant will put his finger on the diagnosis when his juniors have been baffled. This is partly because he is not distracted by details and partly because he may have seen a similar case before. In the same way an experienced family doctor may know whether a patient's symptoms are primarily emotional or physical while a trainee doctor will have to approach the matter step by step.

This factor of experience must be differentiated from the iniquitous "pecking order system" whereby the senior doctor is always right. A mitral diastolic murmur is by definition present when the senior cardiologist can hear it. If the senior cardiologist is a little deaf the murmur does not exist. The junior doctor should, of course, treat his seniors with respect, but respect can be defined as cynicism combined with tact.

2.209 *Much hard work is required by doctors to diagnose obscure disease. If the disease cannot be diagnosed by the senses it must be tracked down by reasoning.*

This is a reiteration of what has been said before. Diagnosing obscure diseases may take a lot of time and hard work and the doctor must be sure that this is time well spent. In other words either the patient will benefit or medical science will be advanced by new information on a rare disease.

Case 19 A man of 52, confined to a mental hospital with presenile dementia, was found to have a low blood sugar. It was mooted whether the dementia was due to chronic or recurrent hypoglycaemia and a complex series of tests was arranged to exclude an insulinoma of the pancreas. These tests proved a nightmare to the staff because it required three people to hold the patient down when blood was taken. The tests were finally abandoned and the patient died peacefully two months later, to the relief of his relatives. This hunt for obscure illness was unjustified because insulinoma is very rare, and although hypoglycaemia can cause brain damage, this damage had already been done and the patient would not have benefited. If an insulinoma had been proven he would probably not have been fit for operation. Anyway, prolongation of life should not have been the primary object in this sad situation.

1.27 *Most doctors are like the pilot of a ship. When the water is calm their mistakes are not noticed but if there is a violent storm everyone will know it is their ignorance that has lost the ship. Any doctor can treat mild illnesses which are far more common than serious disease. The severe illness shows up his lack of skill.*

Harsh words! Either patients are more tolerant today than they used to be or else doctors are better protected by shared responsibility. Serious disease is usually treated in hospital and if there is an error the patient is likely to blame "the hospital". A surgeon is more subject to attack than a physician because when things go wrong they go very wrong and he is, as it were, standing in the open with knife in hand. The physician is hidden somewhere in the cocoon. The family doctor is very much exposed because he is usually alone, but he is protected by being considered an animal of a lower order of intelligence. However he usually has to live with his mistakes because he cannot discharge a patient or family from further attendance.

Not everyone would agree with Hippocrates that "any doctor can treat a mild illness". It could be argued that the trivial and mundane are the true test of a doctor's worth and that "any doctor can become interested in a serious illness but only the best are interested in trivial illness".

1.13 *Just as in all other arts the practitioners of medicine differ greatly in both knowledge and skill.*

This has to be said, although what to do about it is another matter. Factors of intelligence and personality may be unalterable, but laziness, lack of incentive, lack of opportunity to learn, unscrupulousness, a bad system of Medical Care – these are things which can be influenced. Many now fly the flag of "Audit", but audit from outside is difficult to carry out, while self-audit is already done in one way or another by conscientious doctors. It is difficult to design a method of assessing a doctor's work without using compulsion or "snooping" and this, together with its jargon quality, has given the word Audit a bad name. In byegone days, good doctors, like Hippocrates, were known to be good and reaped financial benefits. This is less so nowadays, especially in the British National Health Service where the best paid doctor may be the one who has the largest practice and gives the least time to individual patients. Unfortunately medicine is not like economics where things tend to settle to their own level and customers prefer the "best buy". The customer may have little choice especially if he lives in a place considered unfashionable by doctors.

2.201 *The doctor does his work with a healthy mind and a healthy body. He compares each case with similar cases he has seen in the past, knowing how they were treated and cured.*

This passage stresses two things, the health of the doctor, physical and mental, and his reasoning based on past experience. The juxtaposition of the two may seem odd but I think Hippocrates intended this. A doctor can only reason, as opposed to reacting automatically, if his mind is alert and he can only be alert if he is fit. Hence the enormous benefit to the patient of his doctor playing golf or squash, or having any hobby in which he can become absorbed mentally and physically. A doctor who spends his spare time "glued to the telly" with vacant gaze will probably still have a vacant gaze when he sees his patients next morning and they will know it.

2.199 *Mistakes as well as benefits come from the art of medicine. A thing correctly administered gives benefit, incorrectly given does harm. The art means sometimes being right, sometimes wrong.*

Hippocrates was a humble person, well aware that medicine is a two-edged weapon. Many doctors, past and present, have survived on the assumption they are never wrong. The patient can be wrong, the disease wrong or other doctors wrong. This is a sign of insecurity and lack of wisdom. All doctors find it difficult to take criticism from their colleagues and may become positively enraged by criticism from their patients. Remarks like "Your tablets seem to have made me worse" or "Do you really know what's wrong with me, doctor?" produce spurts of anger in even the most placid. Doctors do not take kindly to patients denying them the attribute of ultimate knowledge. In their calmer moments most doctors have enough insight to realise this attitude is emotional and unreasonable but the spurt of anger is still there. On rare occasions it will become a conflagration which will surprise and alarm the patient who may have made a perfectly sensible and true statement.

2.293 *Remember the different drugs and their properties both simple and complex and carry these in your mind, not on paper. Remember their actions, dose and variability of effect in different cases. This is the beginning, middle and end of therapy.*

Not even Hippocrates would have attained this ideal today because of the multiplicity of the drugs in use, but as Dr

Johnson said, "Knowledge is of two kinds. We know a subject ourselves, or we know where we can find information upon it."

A doctor should divide his armoury of drugs into these two categories. Some he will know and those are the ones he will use frequently. The others he will not know and these he should look up before use. Doing this does not lower him in the patient's esteem. In fact the patient may be impressed that he is getting the very latest in medical care.

The "variability of effect" is especially important in relation to old people, children and those suffering from kidney or liver disease in which excretion or detoxication of the drug may be altered. It is important that the doctor does not blame the patient if he has the misfortune to get severe side effects and even more important that he does not insist on the patient continuing a drug which makes life unbearable for him.

Case 20 A man of 28 attended outpatients with severe hypertension. Various drugs were tried and it was found that the most successful was Ismelin (guanethidine) in combination with a diuretic. The patient suffered hypotensive attacks, sometimes severe enough to make him fall down, and also complained of failure to get an erection during intercourse. He was however cajoled into continuing with the treatment and he was naive and conscientious enough to do so through thick and thin, although he lost first his job and then his wife. The blood pressure readings, as taken in outpatients, were satisfactory and the case was considered a success. This was before the era of more pleasant hypotensive drugs such as B-blockers.

1.317 *Yet some patients ask for what is out of the way and of doubtful benefit. This prejudice deserves to be disregarded but not punished.*

Specially annoying is the patient who asks for something her mother-in-law is taking for similar symptoms or who has read about a new cure in a newspaper or Women's Magazine. Before a doctor gets angry he should remember that when his own car goes wrong he will be the first to tell the motor mechanic what the trouble is and how it should be put right. The mechanic will ignore him and Hippocrates recommends the doctor should ignore the patient's suggestion. However if the treatment is harmless there is no reason why the doctor should not agree provided the patient buys the product herself and does not have it on prescription. The doctor should avoid being talked into giving patent or expensive drugs which he does not consider necessary. This will need determination and tact. A cynic would say that most antibiotics and tranquillisers are in fact prescribed by the patient, the doctor being the propellor of the pen that writes the prescription.

2.297 *Watch your patients carefully because they may not tell you the truth about how they take the medicine you prescribe. Sometimes they die because they do not take what they find disagreeable. There is never a confession and the doctor is blamed.*

It is estimated that nearly half the tablets prescribed under the National Health Service are never actually swallowed by the patient. This usually does not matter and may sometimes be beneficial, but it costs the nation dear and occasionally it costs the patient dear too. If the drug is necessary, for example steroids, digoxin and antibiotics justifiably given, the doctor should issue clear instructions, verbal or written. There is no doubt patients are often untruthful, forgetful or inefficient in taking tablets, but doctors and their families are as bad or worse. A doctor who consults a colleague about illness has almost certainly tried one or two forms of treatment already and is ashamed to mention this. Antibiotics especially are taken in a casual fashion and I knew one doctor who took steroids from time to time for no good reason. So before a doctor gets cross with a patient he should murmur "Mea culpa" to himself.

There is often genuine confusion, especially amongst old people who have a hotch-potch of different coloured tablets in one bottle or, if they are aristocratic, in an ornately carved snuff box. If a doctor visits an old person and finds the drawers crowded with half filled bottles of tablets it is usually a good principle to remove the lot and prescribe vitamin pills.

Case 21 A woman of 89 lived alone but was kept under close observation by neighbours. At times she became confused and twice was admitted to a geriatric hospital, where her condition improved. It was eventually discovered that she had a supply of valium tablets given for "night cramp" which she used to take by the handful, and this caused her confusion and fainting attacks. She now manages well on iron and vitamin tablets.

Case 22 A young woman visited her doctor with vague symptoms which he thought were due to premenstrual tension. He prescribed a diuretic and sleeping tablets. As soon as she got back from the chemist she transferred the tablets to more attractive bottles. Unfortunately she got them the wrong way round and spent a miserable week sleeping all day and going to the toilet all night. She stuck loyally to her treatment but was mildy critical of the doctor when she next saw him.

It appears that Hippocrates felt the doctor should not be blamed for mistakes in treatment. I do not agree with this because few patients take tablets incorrectly on purpose. It is usually because they do not understand, or cannot understand, the instructions they are given. I have heard doctors explaining courses of treatment to elderly patients which are so complex one would almost need a pocket computer to work them out. Failure to assess a patient's intelligence is just as grave an error as prescribing an incorrect dose, and the end result is much the same.

Another common mistake is for a hospital doctor to write to the patient's general practitioner with instructions for treatment without telling the patient to call at the surgery to collect the tablets. When the patient is next seen at the hospital he and his doctor will be criticised for lack of co-operation. I once heard a consultant saying, "These blasted G.P.'s. They don't take a blind bit of notice of my letters." I had not the courage to point out that the lack of communication was his own fault.

1.323 *When an illness is stubborn and the evil grows, in the perplexity of the moment things go wrong. On such occasions one must be bold.*

1.103 *Extreme diseases need extreme treatment.*

The more dangerous the disease the more justifiable it is to give potentially lethal drugs and the doctor should not blame himself too much if death does occur. For example, cytotoxic drugs for conditions such as leukemia must be given largely by trial and error at first until repeated blood counts show what is the correct dose. Even if a careful graph is kept to anticipate a swing towards over-suppression of the marrow, a few patients will die from this. Without treatment virtually all patients would die.

2.199 *The art does not lie only in curing disease by medicines. The greatest physicians cure by general management and everyday substances which no-one would describe as medicine.*

"Everyday substances" are one of the joys of lay medicine and are rarely suggested by a doctor nowadays. A patient would probably be deeply insulted if his doctor advised him to take lemon-and-honey for a cold. He has come for medicine and medicine he must have. So he leaves clutching a prescription for something which is no more effective, probably more dangerous and certainly less fun. This is a pity because a "grandmother's mixture", like home made marmalade, usually tastes better.

We still need Hippocrates' reminder that "the greatest physicians cure by general management". Medicines are not the answer to most illnesses, physical or psychological. The doctor's way of giving (or not giving) a medicine is often as important as the medicine itself. On the assumption that no cough medicines or linctuses, apart perhaps from Linctus Physeptone, are of true scientific value for treating coughs in adults, I usually prescribe the old-fashioned Mist. Expect. This, I explain, must be mixed with two parts of hot water and sipped slowly. If I consider it necessary to prescribe antibiotics as well the patient will probably take them but his faith will be in the medicine. The younger generation are, unfortunately, more sophisticated but folk-memories of "the bottle of medicine" lie deep within us all. I can remember, when I was ill as a child, the doctor giving my mother a bottle of green medicine which I was to be given if my temperature went up. Unfortunately I remained apyrexial so never tasted the medicine, which looked very much like Green Chartreuse.

4.99 *A man's life is short but the art of medicine is long. Opportunity is fleeting, experiment deceptive and judgement difficult. The doctor must be ready not only to do his duty himself but secure the co-operation of the patient, the staff and relatives.*

Doctors have pondered over this for 2,400 years and will continue to ponder. Only one small point will be made. The doctor, whether he works in hospital or family practice, has the duty of "securing the co-operation" of patient, staff and relatives. This implies that although he is a member of a team the ultimate responsibility is his. This does not mean he is necessarily the leader of the team or even, technically speaking, the co-ordinator, but the others must look to him for the final decison. This is what he is trained for and he cannot escape the burden.

5

The Art and the Environment

Hippocrates was fascinated by man's relation to his environment. He was especially interested in the habits of Barbarian races but appears rather gullible over travellers' tales, much more so than his contemporary, Herodotus.

1.125 *The Scythians are a ruddy race because of the cold. The constant jolting of their horses makes them unfit for intercourse. This causes sterility in the men and the women are so fat that the semen cannot enter their bodies.*

How then did the race survive? Hippocrates tell us it was the slave girls who came to the rescue. They were thin enough to have successful intercourse and presumably jolted the menfolk into sexual activity in contradistinction to the horses, who jolted them out of it. The poor Scythians also suffered from iatrogenic impotence. In order to cure joint pains due to excessive riding they underwent the procedure recommended at that time of having the veins behind their ears incised. This led to unfortunate results.

1.129 *After this treatment when the Scythians approach a woman but cannot have intercourse, at first they take no notice and think no more of it. But when two or three or even more attempts are attended with no better success, they think they have sinned against heaven and put on womens' clothes, thinking they have lost their manhood.*

The women-folk also had problems.

1.117 *In the Scythian tribe, the Sauromatae, the women do not lay aside their virginity until they have killed three of their enemies. They have no right breast for while they are yet babies their mothers cauterise it with a red hot bronze instrument constructed for the very purpose.*

A very sensible procedure. These ferocious females needed a free sword arm to reach their target of three victims and attain their heart's desire.

1.111 *Longheads. They consider those with the longest heads to be the noblest so they have the following custom. As soon as the child is born they remodel its head with their hands while it is soft and tender. They they force it to be longer by applying bandages. As time went on the process became natural so that force was no longer needed to lengthen the head.*

It is difficult to fit this in with any known theory of evolution although one is reminded of Weismann's experiment of cutting off the tails of mice to see if they grew shorter in successive generations. Greek philosophers had in fact already worked out the Darwinian theory of evolution by natural selection but had no means of proving it. It could be argued that those female Longheads with naturally longer heads were more seductive, hence they mated early, had more children and the characteristic increased from general to generation.

1.73 *The physician will not, on arrival at a town he does not know, be ignorant of local diseases.*

This referred once more to Hippocrates' advice to be prepared *before* undertaking any task. In smaller western countries there is not much significant variation of illnesses between localities. A doctor who worked in Aberdeen would have no great problems if he moved to Bristol. In larger countries it is more important. Compare Boston and New Orleans, Archangel and Kiev. And even more important when moving from a temperate to a tropic zone when a whole new range of illness presents itself.

1.71 *To study medicine properly in a particular place the doctor must understand the mode of life of the inhabitants, what they like, if they drink heavily, when they eat their meals, whether they are inactive or interested in sport, hardworking, eating much and drinking little. He must also know about the illnesses which are common in that area.*

This is an early statement about community medicine. It is important for a doctor to study the way of life of his patients for two reasons. First he must decide what is normal. For example alcoholism in oil-rig workers is not the same thing as alcoholism in a seaside lodging house in Hastings and "walking" will not mean the same to a London typist as it does to a Scottish ghillie. The second reason is that the doctor should become part of the community and he cannot do this unless he understands the people. He should be able to talk to patients about things that interest them, especially hobbies and sports. For example, in parts of Wales he should know his rugby football and Handel's "Messiah". He should be familiar with his patients' eating habits, whether for example they have high tea or dinner, and what television programmes they are likely to watch. All this may seem trivial but a single inappropriate remark may make the patients feel "he is not one of us" and a close relationship will be that much more difficult.

Strangely enough Hippocrates said little about a patient's job in relation to illness. He had no conception of Industrial Disease as we know it today, apart from the obvious relationship between military service and trauma. The doctor of today is very much aware of such diseases as silicosis and farmer's lung. There are, however, many subtle relationships between work and illness and the following case history is an interesting example.

Case 23 The doctor first saw a child of six called Pamela when she was taking the part of a fairy in "A Midsummer Night's Dream". She danced exquisitely and he mentioned this to her mother who was a patient of his. The mother was pleased and told him they had plans to send Pamela to a ballet school. Pamela in fact had great talent and became quite well known locally as a dancer. She was due to start her full time ballet training at the age of 16, but soon after her fifteenth birthday disaster struck. She started putting on weight and in a matter of months she was so fat that her whole career was in jeopardy. Her mother insisted that she ate no more than anyone else and tried to convince the doctor that the obesity was due to "glands". The doctor doubted this, but because of the seriousness of the situation, sent her to an endocrinologist who could find no abnormality. He remarked in his letter that "Pamela smiles but says nothing". A rigid diet was recommended and this was successful. Pamela lost weight rapidly and showed renewed interest in her dancing. Her manner however remained odd and somewhat detached. Her mother was delighted but later became worried because Pamela was losing too much weight. She was now eating practically nothing and slipped into a state of anorexia nervosa which was intractable. She died of pneumonia at the age of eighteen.

This happened some years ago and much more is known of anorexia nervosa now than it was then. It is probable that Pamela was unable to stand up to the pressures put on her and reacted first by over-eating and later by not eating at all.

What the doctor did not realise at the time was that anorexia nervosa is endemic amongst dancers. If he had known this he might have done something to stop what became an inevitable sequence of events. This was ignorance of an environmental factor.

Knowledge of the locality is important and this is illustrated by the following rare case.

Case 24 Some forty years ago a country doctor, who knew just about all there was to know about his patients, was called in autumn to a cottage where an old man had been found in a state of collapse. This patient was a recluse and somewhat eccentric, wandering round the fields summer and winter. He lived alone but was visited by a niece twice a week. It was she who sent for the doctor. He found the patient in bed, with unpleasant evidence of diarrhoea and vomiting. He was unable to speak and could scarcely move his limbs, which were flaccid. His pulse was slow. The doctor went to the kitchen where he examined a pile of dirty dishes and saucepans. At the bottom of one saucepan was a congealed grey mess. The doctor tasted this by placing a tiny fragment on his tongue. He admitted the patient to hospital as a case of "mushroom" poisoning. He made the diagnosis because twenty years previously he had seen a similar case and he knew that a few fields away there were plentiful mushrooms, but in the middle of the field was a small copse of oak trees and on the edge of the copse grew the pure white toadstool Amanita virosa which is commonly called "The destroying angel" because of its beauty and deadliness. This is the kind of information which, sadly, few family doctors of today possess.

1.183 *It is necessary to consider the patient's mode of life and take it into account when prescribing.*

Paradoxically the chief importance of this statement nowadays relates to the amount of side-effects of the drug which a particular patient can be expected to tolerate. A housewife with hay fever may nod off in her chair after taking antihistamines while a lorry driver may have a fatal accident. A gardener on antidepressants may not plant his row of onions absolutely straight while an accountant may make a serious error leading to financial disaster.

The actual tolerance to drugs is an individual rather than an environmental variation, although customs such as drinking large amounts of alcohol can effect detoxication of some substances. Alcoholics may be difficult to anaesthetise and a man who drinks a bottle of whisky a day will find an ordinary dose of tranquillisers a pin prick. Alcoholism must have been one of the curses of Hippocrates' day and he obviously considered it contributed to many illnesses.

1.285 *. . . in Meliboea a youth took to his bed after for a long time being heated by drunkenness and sexual indulgence.*

Hippocrates observed relationships between the environment and certain diseases but had insufficient evidence to understand why this relationship existed and what to do about it.

1.85 *Those who drink marshy water have always large stiff spleens. In summer there are epidemics of dysentery, diarrhoea and long quartan fevers.*

1.87 *The best streams are those that flow from high places and earthy hills.*

"Long quartan fever" means malaria and Hippocrates incorrectly assumed this was caused by drinking marshy water. He was not aware of the link between marsh-land, mosquitoes and malarial parasites. About four hundred years later Rome, which was a provincial town in his day, controlled malaria by draining the Pontine marshes near the city. This was sensible action based on observation, but it was believed the fever was due to "bad air". The final link was discovered by Ross in 1897, but long before this Cinchona bark had been used as treatment in South America. This is an interesting study of observation as Hippocrates used the word. The results were beneficial even though the theory was incorrect.

2.55 *One must realise that with definite signs or symptoms the bad indicates something bad, the good something favourable whatever the time or place. They have the same significance in Libya as in Delos or Scythia.*

In other words similarities between localities are always greater than differences. The symptoms mean the same and the diseases are usually the same. A man returning by air from a tropical country is more likely to bring back a cold than Lassa fever or other more common tropical illness. But not always . . .

Case 25 A schoolteacher of 50 spent a few days in Kenya supervising examinations. Three weeks after coming home he became feverish and visited his doctor. Examination was normal but, although the patient had been taking prophylactic tablets for malaria, blood was sent as a precaution to the pathology department. No parasites were found. He continued to run an intermittent high fever and because on one occasion crepitations were heard in the lungs he was started on an antibiotic, oxytetracycline. This did not help, so, after a week of fever, he was sent to hospital. The admitting doctor, who had spent some time in India, easily diagnosed malaria on the symptoms, together with signs of minimal jaundice. The patient's own doctor lacked knowledge of this environmental disease because he did not know that some strains of malarial organisms are only partially suppressed by prophylaxis and a single slide may be negative. Anyway prophylaxis should continue for at least six weeks after returning home. The patient recovered rapidly but, since the infection was P. falciparum, the delay in diagnosis could have been serious.

The doctor is handicapped in his dealings with patients because he rarely sees them in their environment. The consulting room is artificial, the patient being expected to conform to an abnormal pattern of behaviour in strange surroundings. The doctor only finds out about the environment by what the patient cares to tell him and this is often a carefully edited version. If an ornithologist were to sit in an office and have birds brought to him in cages he would become very skilled at identifying birds in cages. He would however know little about birds. But how can walking through woods or crawling through marshes be justified in relation to time?

For a similar reason it is understandable that home visits are going out of fashion, but they at least tell the doctor in a few minutes things which would need long and patient discussions to unravel in the consulting room. He may notice the chaos of the home where the mother has "given up", the weeds in the garden, the unmade beds upstairs, the over-meticulous cleanliness of the obsessive housewife and, most of all, the concealed or overt hostility between members of the family. In the consulting room a mother will not scream at her child or hit him. In the home she may do so, or at least make as if to do so. This the doctor will notice. His visit is even more useful if he arrives unexpectedly. The way to find out how an obese patient is dieting is to call in at dinner time. The doctor may glimpse a plate loaded with steak and potatoes being rushed to the kitchen.

A doctors' practice recently decided to change their system of visiting. Instead of all the doctors doing a morning surgery then starting their calls at about 11 a.m., one doctor each day did an early morning round starting at 8.30 a.m. Quite often he found the patient had gone out shopping with the intention of putting herself in bed and "being ill" before the doctor arrived later in the day. This caused a lot of embarrassment. One patient was not at home because he was driving home from holiday, yet the doctor's receptionist was told he was unfit to attend surgery. Cases have been recorded where the patient has come to the surgery herself to say she's not fit to come to the surgery. This is the other side of the coin, illustrating that some patients who ask for a home visit could easily come to the surgery. In time the doctor or receptionist will come to recognise these families and try to convert them to a more reasonable attitude.

Case 26 A married woman of forty attended the doctor frequently because of headaches. No cause could be found for these and they did not respond to simple treatment. He tried to get her to talk about herself but she denied all anxiety and spoke at length about trivial matters. On one occasion he was called to the house when she had influenza. While examining her he heard someone laughing in the next room. When he remarked on this the patient became upset. It turned out that she was looking after her senile mother who was demented and incontinent. She had been ashamed to mention this but finally broke down and wept. Her headaches improved when the doctor showed sympathy he really felt and provided help. It is interesting that on going through the front door he had been puzzled because the house was excessively tidy but *smelt of urine*. It is possible that many patients have "skeletons in the cupboard". This is sometimes called the Jane Eyre Syndrome because in Charlotte Brontë's book the mad wife was secretly kept locked in the attic but gave the game away by eerie night wanderings and occasional bursts of demoniac laughter.

Hippocrates showed personal interest in his patients. We know this because he wrote of them as individuals, often assuming that the reader, being part of the same community, would know whom he was talking about.

1.179 *There were two cases of suppuration, both fatal; Ciatistonax who lived near the temple of Heracles and the serving maid of Seymus, the fuller.*

Hippocrates spent most of his time in fairly small communities, Athens being an exception, and we can imagine that, like the country doctor described earlier in this chapter, he knew what was going on. He would meet his patients in their true environment, the street, the market place, the theatre, and he probably knew Ciatistonax and Seymus before he was called to their homes. Aristotle defined the ideal city as one where everyone knew everyone else by sight. Nowadays this could not be said of a village let alone a town or city.

However, a family doctor in a town or village may learn a lot by observing what is going on, from his car window in particular. Illness, or lack of it, may be noticed or assessed, for example a patient with Parkinsonism, a "cardiac case" walking briskly down the road, or the old man with emphysema who was not dyspnoeic in the surgery but is seen hanging on to a lamp post to get his breath.

Case 27 A patient in the building trade attended the surgery with a strained back. On examination there was pain on full flexion. The patient was advised to stay away from work and rest. Three days later, while travelling past the patient's house the doctor noticed him on the roof repairing the tiles. The doctor made a point of stopping the car and shouting up at him to ask him how his back was. The patient was surprised and maintained his balance with some difficulty. He went back to work next day. This appeared to be a true case of malingering which is not very common.

Even more important is the way people *behave* when they think they are not being watched. The "devoted" mother is seen slapping her child, the subjugated wife is seen walking an exact three paces behind her husband, the henpecked husband carries the baby *and* the shopping.

Case 28 A middle aged businessman had been attending the doctor with pains in the chest. He was a very extrovert man who always called the doctor "Squire" and pressed invitations on him to "drop round and have a glass of whisky". His heartiness was irritating. One afternoon the doctor caught sight of the patient's reflection in a shop window. He was obviously extremely depressed, and being unobserved, as he thought, had allowed his mask to slip. At the next consultation the doctor spent half an hour gently leading him to talk about his worries. He was, in fact, seriously troubled by guilt about sexual deviation and was contemplating suicide. He might well have done this had it not been for a chance observation in the "environment" rather than the surgery.

Sometimes by putting patients together in groups a social environment can be created. Unfortunately this too makes for a highly artificial situation. The patients sit in a circle and talk or listen so that the garrulous become more garrulous and the shy more frustrated in their shyness. The magic word "Group" is losing its magic because it suggests artificially mixed immiscible substances. A good group leader can sometimes work the miracle. On the other hand patients who mix as friends in both general and mental hospitals help each other greatly by forming natural groups. As Hippocrates pointed out, the doctor should work with Nature, and not against it, and interference in relationships may be just as damaging as interference in physical illness.

He was of course helped by the small size of the population he was dealing with because this formed natural groups which related directly to their environment.

1.175 *About the equinox up to the setting of the Pleiades and during winter there was much illness. The patients who died were chiefly striplings, young people, people in their prime, the smooth, the fair-skinned, the straight-haired, the black-haired, the black-eyed, those who had lived recklessly and carelessly, the thin-voiced, the rough-voiced, the lispers, the passionate.*

Hippocrates was interested in the relationship between the seasons and illness and would record carefully the time of year and the weather conditions preceding each epidemic and its later effect. Nowadays, we tend to ignore the effects of the weather because we can usually protect ourselves from it. Hippocrates gave it priority.

1.71 *Whoever wishes to pursue properly the science of medicine must proceed thus. First he ought to consider what effects each season of the year can produce.*

He especially noted the dangers of Spring, a time when, we would suppose, the queues of gloomy patients at the surgery would get shorter, but in fact the suicide rate increases. "April is the cruellest month."

4.129 *In Spring occurs melancholia, madness, epilepsy. . . .*

1.255 *In all the cases described Spring was the worst enemy and caused most deaths.*

Hippocrates considers diet very important and, long before the advent of electrocardiograms and cholesterol levels, he made the following observation:

4.119 *Fat people are liable to die suddenly.*

And here are two general statements about geriatrics:

4.133 *Old men suffer from shortness of breath, catarrh and coughing, difficulty in passing water, joint pains, kidney disease, giddiness, strokes, loss of weight, generalised pruritus, sleeplessness, watery discharge from the bowels, eyes and nostrils, short sightedness, cataracts, and deafness.*

1.101 *Old men have blockages because of the flabbiness and wasting of their blood vessels, so that some die suddenly and others become paralysed either on the right or left.*

Hippocrates noted that many illnesses followed overindulgence in food and other things.

1.31 *A man who eats a heavy lunch becomes sluggish in body and mind and falls a prey to yawning, drowsiness and thirst . . . however, a man who misses his lunch becomes weak, trembly and faint. His stomach seems to "hang" and he becomes listless and depressed. It depends on which he is used to.*

Even in Hippocrates' time it seems that men were so "civilised" that they were dependent on the habit of regular meals. The above passage could refer to a businessman's lunch of today or, contrariwise, what happens when he decides to work through his lunch hour. Primitive man, the predator, ate where and when he could and was in many ways better for it. Civilised man is a slave to custom and slavery has its disadvantages, one of which is inability to adapt. Hippocrates anticipated Darwin in the following remarkable passage about primitive man.

1.19 *Many and terrible were the sufferings of men from strong and brutish living . . . the majority naturally perished having too weak a constitution, while the stronger resisted longer.*

He goes on to describe the evolution of cooking and agriculture to counteract this "brutish living" and unsuitable diet. However, man always has and always must compete with his environment to be healthy in body and mind.

1.137 *Where the land is rich, soft and well watered the inhabitants are fleshy, inarticulate, lazy and generally cowardly in character. Laziness and sleepiness are observed in them and as far as the arts are concerned they are thick-witted. But where the land is bare, waterless, rough, oppressed by storms in winter and burnt by the sun in summer, there you will see men who are hard, lean, articulate, upright in posture and hairy. Their natures are energetic, vigilant, stubborn and independent, wild rather than placid, of more than average sharpness and intelligence in the arts and more than average courage in war.*

This is something of a generalisation especially as far as "intelligence in arts" is concerned. Nowadays we tend to associate culture with large cities and towns, that is to say "well watered" places. It must be remembered that Hippocrates lived just after the Greek–Persian wars when the hardy West defeated the indolent East and this must have coloured his outlook. At this time Greek art of all forms was intensely creative and history shows that small states under military attack often produce bursts of artistic activity. Athens was the greatest example of all time, but think also of the Normans who set a fashion in conquest and church building while Elizabethan England defeated the Armada and produced Shakespeare and Bacon.

1.115 *When men are not independent and their own masters but are organised by others, they lack enthusiasm for military service. Fatigue, death and separation from their families are only for the aggrandisement of their masters. But if they are independent they run risks for their own sakes, receiving the reward of bravery and the penalty of cowardice.*

Substitute the word "work" for "military service" and this passage should give food for thought to economists and politicians of our own time. People who work for themselves and their own families bear hardships which they would not dream of putting up with if they worked for an organisation, and of course the larger the organisation the less the tolerance of the individual to hard work. Hippocrates would have approved of Schumaker's interesting book "Small is Beautiful". As the title suggests, Schumaker puts forward the theory that small units are not only happier and less wasteful but sometimes more productive than large industrial concerns of the conveyor belt type. This has a bearing on medicine in two ways. First, people who work for themselves, who know the other people they work with, who see the end product of their labours, tend to be happier and therefore healthier than those who are submerged in a massive organisation. Second, a small medical unit is happier and more efficient than an outsize one. This can be seen in hospitals where the contented people are to be found in small groups away from the main stream, and where the old system of a ward being under the charge of a single ward sister, even if she was a battle-axe, usually worked much better than the present multi-unit system with nebulous authority.

In general practice the surgery is the base for about twenty people who work together with the same end in view and who all know each other and meet frequently. A large health centre may lose this quality. In professional life a person rarely quarrels with someone he meets face to face. Over the telephone or with postal correspondence it is a different matter. Departments bear malice towards each other through lack of personal contact.

1.115 *With regard to the lack of spirit and courage amongst the inhabitants, the reason why they are less warlike and more gentle in character is the uniformity of the seasons. For there occur no mental shocks or violent physical change which are more likely to steel the temper and impart to it fierce passion than monotonous sameness.*

Again we have to translate the rather militaristic attitude of Hippocrates to the social attitudes of today. War is considered undesirable and rightly so but this is only a recent phenomenon. From Marathon to Trafalgar, from Agincourt to Dunkirk it has been a mainspring of energy which we now lack. Sport and industrial competition are poor substitutes. The glory of the Russian worker who produces more ball-bearings than his fellow workers is not quite on a par with the glory of the heroes of Greece and Troy.

1.133 *For uniformity engenders slackness while variation engenders endurance in both body and soul. Rest and slackness are food for cowardice, endurance and exertion for bravery. Independent people taking risks on their own behalf and not on behalf of others are willing and eager to go into danger for they themselves enjoy the prize of victory.*

If we apply the second sentence to the patient visiting the doctor we land ourselves in the debate as to whether it is an advantage to be responsible for one's own medical care. Is it better to pay for medical services, that is to say to *earn* them, even if part can be claimed back? Or is it better to accept them as a right in a welfare state? In general terms we nowadays tend to attach little value to things that are free because money has become a standard of value. It does not need a philosopher to point out the fallacy of this because most of the things of true value, the sky above, the world around, relationship with others, are free and if we encumber them with money we in fact decrease their worth. It is the tragedy of advanced civilisation that strife has to be seen in monetary or military terms, but this must be accepted as a fact, not however necessarily an unalterable fact. Not to strive is to become slack and cowardly, and the patient who absorbs care, medical or social, is depriving himself of necessary stimuli. Arthur Hugh Clough's tenth commandment was:

"Thou shalt not covet, but tradition
Approves all forms of competition."

6

The Art and Self Reliance

2.7 *But men in fact do die, some because of the serverity of the disease before they call the doctor, others dying immediately after, living a day or a little longer, before the doctor by his art can combat the disease.*

This stresses the need to call the doctor early because only he can treat the illness correctly, or so it is supposed.

Hippocrates belonged to the Aesculapian guild, a band of doctors who originated from temple priests. They were a closed shop and very much dependent on mystique for their survival, and, of course, this mystique has been handed down to the present day, although now it is related to science rather than religion. In fact it predated Hippocrates by many thousand years since the first known record of a "doctor" is a cave-painting in southern France which portrays a figure riddled with mystique in the form of an ugly mask and horns on the head. It was necessary for the Aesculapiads to consider that they and they only could understand the art of medicine and that lay people were ignorant and interfering. Hippocrates himself leant in this direction although he gave laymen some credit.

2.63 *Even a layman could correctly describe some individual diseases by carefully asking a patient his experiences.*

Notice the disparaging word "even". Hippocrates felt the value of laymen in medicine was in the information they could provide for the doctor, rather than their own ideas of diagnosis and treatment.

1.315 *Do not hesitate to enquire of laymen if thereby there seems likely to result any improvement in treatment.*

He was particularly critical of the layman's assessment of both doctors and medicine.

2.67 *Laymen do not accurately distinguish doctors who are excellent but rather praise or blame strange remedies. . . . Ordinary folk show their most stupid side so that quacks get the reputation of being physicians.*

Again the traditional attack of proper doctors on the non-professionals. The same idea was put across rather more strongly and with superb alliteration by John Hall, an English surgeon, in 1565 A.D.:

> "Whereas there is one Surgeon apprenticed to his Art and one Physician that has travelled in the true study and exercise of Physic, there are ten that are presumptious smearers, smatterers and abusers of the same; yea, smiths, cutlers, carters, cobblers, carriers of leather, carpenters and a great rabble of women."

In Hippocrates' day the doctor would be summoned only in the event of severe illness, except perhaps by rich people who, then as now, looked upon medicine as a hobby which they could afford to indulge in. It must be remembered that only in the last few decades has a doctor been considered the first port of call and I hope to show that even today this is far from the truth. Throughout the ages the chief standby has been the mother of the household, who was the traditional dispenser of medicines, helped by neighbours, friends and possibly a local wise-woman.

Round about 1400 A.D. Chaucer wrote:

> "Wel may the sike man biwaille and wepe,
> There as ther nye no wyf the house to kepe."

and in one of the first medical surveys on record, which was conducted by Bishop Wren in 1660, the villagers of Dry Drayton near Cambridge declared, "None practice physic nor professeth midwifery but charitably one neighbour helpeth another".

The Hippocratic Collection consisted of medical treatises and unfortunately gave no record of home treatment apart from peculiar customs of Barbarian tribes. I intend to follow Hippocrates' precepts on self-reliance and independence into this field, because people are just beginning to realise its importance.

1.133 *Independent people taking risks on their own behalf and not on behalf of others are willing and eager to go into danger, for they themselves enjoy the prize of victory.*

2.279 *Alertness and exercise of intellect bring with them something that helps to make life beautiful.*

Some years ago I came to the conclusion that most patients who came to see me had already been extensively diagnosed and treated. Even in a so-called free medical service it was usual for people to try their own hand first, either because they wanted to or because they did not wish to trouble the doctor. It was part of their family life and culture to take their own remedies, whether these originated from grandmother or a "T.V. advert". To say this made life more beautiful would be an exaggeration but it made it more fun.

To test this in a scientific way, that is to say with Hippocratic observation, I asked a thousand patients who came to my surgery what sort of treatment they had received before coming to see me. Who had advised treatment? Was it good or bad treatment? Had they accepted the advice? A statistical account of this survey was published in the Journal of the Royal College of General Practitioners of May 1973. (23.255).

It was not entirely surprising to find that only 4% had come to the doctor as first choice, the others having received advice from elsewhere or treated themselves. It is, therefore, something of a mockery to call the doctor a primary care physician because he is providing secondary care in nearly every case.

The tiny group of independents consisted mainly of sad people, the widowed, the separated, the solitary or those who had diseases so terrible, they thought, that they could disclose it to no-one but a doctor.

Case 29 A middle-aged man came to the surgery complaining of backache. He had recently lost his wife and had consulted no-one because he "had no friends and anyway if I got some ointment there's no-one to rub it in for me now".

Case 30 A woman in her forties came to the doctor with a lump in her breast. She had noticed this six months before but had kept it secret, even from her husband. The doctor tried to find out why she had done this and she insisted it was not because she was afraid of cancer but because it was "not nice". Fortunately it turned out to be a cyst.

Of the other 96% some had had one piece of advice, some many. The average was 2·3 consultations before visiting the doctor, the record being a boy with acne who had tried eleven different forms of treatment. It seemed that skin conditions, being easily seen and not usually serious, were open to all sorts of suggestions. People with sociable jobs were also likely to get plenty of advice.

Case 31 A married village shop-keeper had a persistent cough. She received advice from her husband, an ex-matron, a doctor's receptionist and five customers, of whom three recommended Golden Syrup, one boiled onion gruel and one the application of a hot brick.

It is interesting that golden syrup, the modern version of treacle, is a very old remedy indeed. It was used by the Aesculapiads before the time of Hippocrates and is mentioned throughout the ages, in particular by Chaucer and the 17th century diarist John Evelyn who never travelled abroad without his bottle of treacle. Another Aesculapian medicine Hiera Picra, the holy remedy, survived in various formulations and was last heard of in the market place of Birmingham in 1929 where it was sold as Pickery Sticks.

Where did patients in this survey obtain advice? The majority were almost equally divided between those who bought or prepared remedies off their own bat, those who sought advice from a friend or neighbour, those who discussed it with their spouse and those who approached some other relative. Less commonly, information was obtained from books, magazines and television or from chemists and friends with nursing experience.

The soundness of advice was difficult to measure but my own assessments were checked by six other doctors independently and the agreement was close. It showed, as expected, that chemists and nurses gave the best advice, although nurses sometimes scared the wits out of their friends. All other categories were much the same except that impersonal sources of advice, such as books, magazines and T.V., came low on the list. Hippocrates considered that when self-treatment was good this was by luck rather than judgement, but we cannot accept this now if we agree that some categories of lay people give better advice than others.

2.197 *I believe it is possible to profit by the art of medicine without calling a doctor, not by knowing what is correct or incorrect treatment, but by chance to employ self-treatment which the doctor would have prescribed.*

Of the relatives, wives gave the best advice and mothers-in-law and mothers the worst, although this was probably a reflection of their relationship with the daughters-in-law and daughters who resented interference. Husbands rarely gave practical advice but liked to opt out and say, "You had better go to the doctor". In fact men, as a whole, were reluctant to give advice while women appeared to consider it their duty and a source of pleasure. A typist in an office who said she had a headache brought work to a standstill while the staff discussed "what auntie said", articles in a recent women's magazine and the relative merit of tablets advertised on T.V. A mechanic in a garage who made a similar remark received no advice but a few ribald comments such as "Go and jump in the river" or "What were you up to last night?" It seems men do not take these things as seriously as women, and in the survey it was exceedingly rare for men to ask or receive advice from another man.

The commonest impersonal sources of advice were home-doctor books and women's magazines, followed by newspapers and television, and 16% of advice was from one or the other.

Women's magazines gave a lot of information, on average seventeen articles or advertisements in each issue. Some of these were cosmetic rather than medical. For example one magazine showed an advertisement on "how to reduce the waist-line by nine inches in three days". In the same issue was another advertisement on "How I increased my bust line from 34 inches to 39 inches in just eight weeks". A combination of these two would have been interesting and is reminiscent of the Scythian "longheads" already referred to who also sought beauty by artificial means.

Home doctor books were usually out of date and sometimes had pride of place on the book shelf with a bible and an equally out of date dictionary. The average (median) age was 27·5 years. One old lady used a book dated 1894 which she claimed had been instrumental in "saving five lives". Another used a medical work by Aristotle who was born about the time Hippocrates died. Most were badly written and easily misunderstood, although since the survey was carried out some excellent home-care books have been published.

Case 32 A girl of 19 consulted her doctor about an itchy rash. She had already looked at a twenty-year-old medical dictionary and rightly came to the conclusion she had scabies. The treatment recommended was "sulphur and hot baths" but she had in fact borrowed some benzoyl benzoate application from a friend. She had thus had the correct diagnosis and treatment. However, the medical dictionary had included an illustration of a greatly magnified scabies mite. The patient was having nightmares about these giant shrimp-like creatures burrowing into her skin. Her anxiety had reached phobic proportions and was much more difficult to treat than the original scabies.

This was an example of harmful advice due to misunderstanding and anxiety. Bad advice was relatively uncommon. It could cause an upset in various ways – excess anxiety (60), incorrect treatment (49), harmful delay (7) and unnecessary expense (6). To get things in perspective, we must look at the assessments for soundness of all self care or advice in the thousand patients involved in the survey.

Good or complete	48%
Slightly helpful	35%
Harmless	11%
Harmful	5%

In other words, according to doctors, who have an expert but one-sided view of these matters, most self care is beneficial to a greater or lesser extent and about half was considered good. The doctor's cold cure is probably no more effective than the patient's cold cure, and his analgesic tablets are much the same as the aspirin from the cupboard. A "harmless" remedy is satisfactory if the disease is self limiting and Hippocrates accepted that in some cases Nature was more important than treatment.

2.289 *In fact, although doctors take many things in hand, many diseases are also overcome for them spontaneously.*

It is more informative to study the relatively few "harmful" cases, although this may give an unsympathetic impression of lay medicine.

Case 33 A hairdresser of 23, while setting a nurse's hair, felt a little giddy. She mentioned this to the nurse who said,

"You know what that is? Blood pressure!" The hairdresser was worried and finally summoned up courage to see her doctor. The blood pressure was normal and she was told the giddiness was due to standing for a long time in a hot room.

Case 34 A man of 69 had noticed a sore place on his forehead some ten years before visiting the surgery. It had got slowly bigger and his wife had repeatedly suggested he should see a doctor. Finally he went to a herbalist who undertook a course of treatment with ointments and medicine "through the blood stream", over a period of three years. The lesion continued to grow and the patient tried zinc ointment. Although his wife and various friends pressed him to see a doctor it was a chemist who finally persuaded him to go. He was found to have a classical rodent ulcer, one and a half inches in diameter, with rolled edges. This responded to radiotherapy. He died two years later from a different illness.

Case 35 A good-looking married woman of 26 was worried because her breasts were too small. One friend advised exercises while another told her not to wear a bra. A nursing friend recommended exercises. These suggestions did not help so she began to spend money – a tube of cream (£2.00) from an advertisement in a woman's magazine, cream and tablets (£3.50) from another woman's magazine and £20 for a course of exercises at a beauty clinic. She had to admit that she was no better off at the end of it all. She was reassured that a pretty face and small breasts was better than an ugly face and large breasts.

The following case illustrates the remarkable suggestive power of the media.

Case 36 A young married woman attended the surgery complaining of rather vague abdominal symptoms. She looked anxious and after the doctor had carried out an examination which was negative, he tried to get to the bottom of the matter. It turned out that she was markedly similar in appearance to the internationally famous British athlete, Lilian Board, who died of cancer at an early age. After watching a television programme

> showing Lilian Board in the late stages of her illness she began to experience symptoms of the kind associated with cancer of the bowel. She admitted all this but it took a lot of reassurance and listening before the symptoms disappeared. Two other patients, both of a similar age and blondes, came to the surgery with an almost identical history. Each had identified herself with Lilian Board. It is, of course, common for patients to take upon themselves the symptoms of seriously ill or dead relatives, and illness of a well-loved character in a television serial has the same effect. After all they are one of the family.

Household remedies, or as Hippocrates put it,

2.199 *. . . everyday substances which no-one would account as medicines . . .*

made up 14·6% of all items of treatment. They were more commonly used in rural areas, by the old, as one would expect, and by teenagers as one would not expect. Perhaps there is a link between granddaughters and grandmothers during the period of rebellion against parents. The daughter does not do what mother says but goes to grannie and uses her remedy.

The remedies used were a fascinating assortment and some were the same as those mentioned by Hippocrates. It is interesting that such things as honey, alcohol, lemon, onions and vinegar have universal healing properties and are effective on various parts of the anatomy. Onion, for example, is used as onion gruel for colds; it soothes insect bites; the soft centre portion is extracted and inserted in the ear to stop earache.

Alcohol of various sorts is popular, both as an internal remedy, for example whisky and milk for colds, or an external application. Hot blackcurrant juice is another cold remedy and dandelion and burdock wine is given for depression. The list is endless and if the reader feels faintly amused by these old customs it must be pointed out that on average one patient out of three in this survey had used household remedies before coming to the doctor. Many more had used chemist's remedies like aspirin, often from the family store-cupboard.

Hippocrates would have been interested in all this, but disappointed that magic, of the kind he disapproved of, is still extensively used. Some of this is modern magic, such as copper rings for rheumatism or even "magnetic bracelets with six built-in magnets worn by millions of delighted users". I might also mention the magic of the television screen where the furrowed brow of the young housewife is instantly soothed out by her favourite headache tablet, making her into a Helen of Troy. Since all women would like to lose their headaches and become Helen of Troy, the magic works. Traditional magic may be dying out but it was frequently mentioned, often in a shamefaced manner, suggesting that patients did even odder things than they were willing to admit to.

Case 37 A married woman of 22 had recurrent styes in the eye for two months. She applied Golden Eye Ointment and later, on the chemist's advice, a proprietary eye ointment. A magazine article suggested general cleanliness was the most important factor. The patient's father suggested she applied a wedding ring to the eye twice a day.

The association of "gold" and eye disease can be traced back to Greek times. In the city of Bath there is an engraved stone advertising a special golden eye lotion dating to the Roman occupation. Golden Eye Ointment is in the line of descent and the wedding ring treatment is in common use in the Midlands of England. One patient stated, "It is better to use the wedding ring of a newly married couple. It is more potent."

Case 38 An unmarried girl of 31 complained of chilblains. Friends recommended two advertised products and calcium tablets. A neighbour suggested she sat with her feet in the toilet. When the doctor showed surprise he was told, "It goes back donkeys' years". He mentioned this interesting piece of information to the next patient in the surgery and she was annoyed that he found it amusing. She used the same treatment herself. It is in fact commonly used, although for children chamber-pots are preferred, but these are now becoming unfashionable except as articles of antique value.

Case 39 A bachelor of 38 became depressed. He was afraid to go to the doctor but consulted a medical dictionary from which he learnt nothing useful. When he mentioned his depression to a friend he was told it was "due to the moon". He was advised to stay indoors when the moon was full. He found this advice helpful and even after he had been treated with antidepressants he always "felt poorly when the moon was full". Cyclical illness in relation to the moon is not as absurd as it sounds. Many creatures regulate their sexual functions "by the light of the moon" and the jump between hormonal and mental disturbances is a small one.

Many other similar cases could be described. Warts in particular have mystical attributes because of their resistance to medical treatment followed by a sudden mysterious disappearance. Just as the Greeks looked for a reason for everything patients today must seek a reason for their warts disappearing. By coincidence some charm or special remedy may have been used shortly before; if not they may have done something out of the ordinary, like eating tinned crab or asparagus or spilling tomato ketchup on their fingers. They tell their friends, who rather shamefacedly start smearing tomato ketchup on their warts. One patient in the survey used the age-old method of touching the wart with a piece of raw beef which was then buried in the garden at the stroke of midnight. Hippocrates would have smiled at this. Have not warts become a divine disease as epilepsy was in his day?

2.139 *It is no more sacred than any other disease but has a natural cause. Its supposed sacredness is due to man's ignorance and his wonder at its unusual character.*

These magical remedies are exciting to read about and fulfil a need not provided for by packaged scientific treatment. These needs should be recognised and not necessarily discouraged. They must, however, be seen as a small part of household remedies, which are mostly mundane and themselves only a small part of all self care. And self care must be seen as a part of total medical care. What in fact do people do when they are ill?

The answer is given in the diagram below, which was compiled by the Panel on Self Care, showing actions taken by those suffering from symptoms.

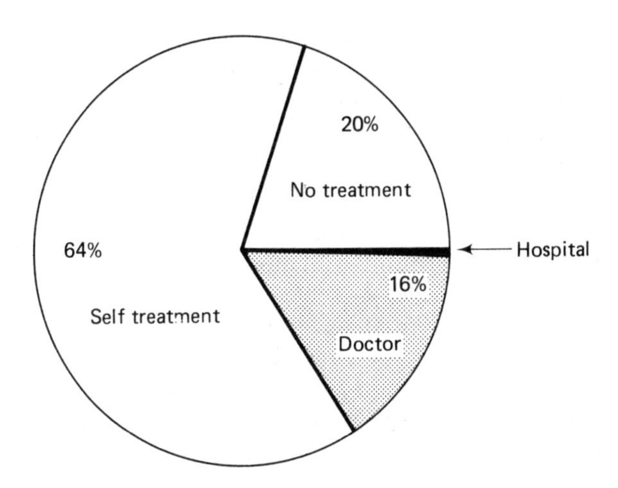

This dial, as we will call it, represents the action people take for the entire range of illness from the trivial to the catastrophic. The narrow dark segment (16%) represents people going to the doctor and the rather thick line (1%) people going to hospital. The smaller white segment (20%) represents people who do nothing but are prepared to ride it out. The large segment (64%) represents self treatment with chemist's or household remedies.

It is worth while pondering over this dial. To most patients the dark segment is a refuge which they enter when the need is pressing, although each person has a different definition of what is "pressing". It may be a cold or it may be terminal cancer.

To many doctors the dark segment is the beginning and end of medicine, the rest representing matters which are trivial and unscientific. The Aesculapiads of Greece would have agreed wholeheartedly with this because they had to, for reasons of prestige and finance. We hope that Hippocrates was a little more tolerant. Lord Beveridge, the forerunner of the National Health Service, believed that this segment could be enlarged in a "free and comprehensive medical service" with doctors available to all. In this way illness would become less and the government could budget for decreasing costs as the years went by. This turned out to be "a miscalculation of sublime proportions", as Enoch Powell described it.

To some hospital doctors, and I hope they are a dying race, the dark segment is itself trivial, medicine beginning and ending in their narrow 1% line. What went on before the patient is admitted to hospital or attends a clinic is already past history.

Illich looks upon the dark segment as something rather sinister. Like the hand of a clock the lower edge of the segment is stealthily creeping round until most of the dial will be blacked out by the "medicalisation of life". It is an insatiable monster creating more and more illness to keep its servants in employment and consuming an ever increasing proportion of the national income. Self care has been made into a felony by the medical profession, because it does not suit their ideas or their pockets. A few people of deep and sincere religious conviction believe the segment to be evil in its own right, an affront to God.

Politicians and economists fear this dark segment. If only it could be made a little bit smaller, perhaps 10% or even 15%, they would sleep more soundly at night. There would be money to spend in making the service better or improving other equally important services such as education. Yet there is always pressure on them to enlarge the segment. Illness must be hunted down by screening techniques, so the disease is treated as soon as it begins or even before, which follows the Hippocratic aphorism:

2.211 *If the disease and treatment start together the disease will not win the race.*

Standards of health must be forever improving until the only person who is abnormal is the one who is convinced he is fit. We see this already. When a mother has a baby she is unlikely to have a normal delivery. Even if she thinks it is the doctors probably will not agree. As for the baby, it will have to be very clever to avoid being put on an "at risk" register by some person for some reason. An exaggeration? Yes, but not much of one.

Like the Greeks we should fall back on reason and recognise each of these opinions as a partial truth. We should also sit back and make some assumptions so that at least we have a working basis on which to plan medical care.

The first assumption is that modern medicine has brought benefits to man that have far exceeded any disadvantages. Only a fool would deny this.

The second is that the medical establishment has outrun itself economically and culturally. It is a child in an adult world.

The third is that most of its faults are due to greed, intolerance, selfishness, dogmatism or mere incompetence and some of these could be put right.

Where do we start? With the patient of course, because he is, to use an expression I detest but which is in fact accurate, "what medicine is all about".

4.59 *A wise man should consider that health is the greatest of human blessings and should learn by his own thought to derive benefit in his illness.*

These words should make us pause because they are fundamental. The illness starts fair and square with the patient. It is his property and he must decide what to do with it. First he must make up his mind if he should even permit himself to be ill by the recognised methods of telling someone else about it, taking an aspirin or seeing a doctor. The doctor hopefully will do what the patient wants; that is to say he will give his official blessing if the patient really is ill or wishes to be; or he will reassure him if he is not ill or does not wish to be. If the doctor says the wrong thing there is trouble and this itself may lead to illness. But whatever he says the final decision is the patient's.

Case 40 The Brontë family, who lived at Howarth Rectory in Yorkshire in the early nineteenth century, were stricken with tuberculosis. Neither Branwell nor his sister Emily wanted medical attention in their last illness and Emily never saw a doctor at all. Branwell insisted on dying in a standing position which, after a painful struggle, he succeeded in doing. Emily continued knitting until three hours before death and only stopped because she could no longer see. "No coward soul is mine", she had written in one of her last poems. We might call this obstinacy but nowadays it would be nothing short of stupidity, because they could have been treated with streptomycin or some more modern antibiotic and not to see a doctor would have been "suicidal". But at the time they were doing the right thing, for them, because as Hippocrates put it,

1.267 . . . *nothing would do them any good.*

The present day equivalent of consumption is untreatable cancer and, provided the patient knows what he is up to, he has a right to do what the Brontës did, although he would be unlikely to carry it out in such a heroic fashion. Illich complains that "hospital death is now endemic" and a patient who puts his foot on the bottom rung of the ladder of hospital investigation usually has to climb to the top however dizzy it may make him. Once his sights are set on the hospital he will probably end by dying there, treated with as much care and skill the staff have time for. "No-one is allowed to die without being cured."

For a patient self-care may be the most appropriate form of help provided he does not suffer from a condition that must be treated by a doctor, which in fact comprises only a small proportion of total illness. This includes conditions which require surgery, infections which require antibiotics (a minority) and things like cardiac failure where life may be prolonged with the patient remaining in comparative comfort. Self-limiting illnesses should not be the doctor's province unless he can provide symptomatic relief which a patient cannot obtain for himself, such as for example severe pain. Again this is relatively uncommon. Mental illness is a subject in its own right.

Recently Marsh, an English family doctor, has taken this point. He put up a notice in his surgery, backed by the Health Authority, stating that Patent Medicines would no longer be issued to patients. After an initial near-riot the practice settled down to providing care for those who needed it with more time for individual patients. Those with coughs, colds and trivial complaints bought or made their own remedies and were probably better for it. No doubt a few could not manage without repeated support from their doctor.

This brings us to the contradiction which the reader has been burning to point out. How does the patient know his illness is not serious unless he sees a doctor? Or, putting it another way, a patient must visit a doctor to be sure there is no need for him to visit a doctor. This is the sort of dilemma the Greeks loved to discuss.

Being faced with a dilemma is like being faced with a charging bull. You have a choice of being impaled on either the left horn or the right horn – hence the expression "horns of a dilemma" – unless you can think of a way out of it. The dilemma here is that either more patients should see the doctor so that serious illness will be diagnosed early or that less patients should see the doctor so that he should have more time and facilities to diagnose serious illness earlier.

Various solutions offer themselves. First, to have more doctors. This would make the economist and Illich have nightmares. Apart from being too expensive it is self-defeating. As readers of "Small is Beautiful" or people who have worked in a hospital will know, the more doctors you have the less work each will do. In a provincial hospital in Britain the junior staff may have increased by about four times but the output will have increased very little. Methods of diagnosis and treatment have improved but this is not in the main a reflection of the numbers of doctors.

The second choice is to accept a higher morbidity and death rate as inevitable, a fatalistic attitude which may become reality.

Thirdly, we could depend more on "sub-doctors" who are cheaper to train. This is now becoming a world wide practice. Examples are the barefoot doctors of China who with standard knowledge and standard equipment can cope with most illness, the *feltschauer* of Russia, medical assistants in the U.S.A., and those health visitors or nurses in Britain who have increased responsibilities. These latter are still treated with some suspicion by doctors and the nursing authorities who believe that nurses should know their place. It should be obvious that, provided their tasks are defined, they will learn to do them far better than doctors who are meant to know everything about everything. Who in their senses would want a family doctor to bandage their sore thumb or deliver their baby? Who in an Intensive Care Unit would prefer a junior doctor to an experienced staff nurse? It is interesting that in some African countries the number of doctors is intentionally limited, reliance being placed on peasants with a modicum of training. This should work very well because, by and large, tropical diseases have a standard presentation and treatment.

The fourth way out of the dilemma is for people to understand and treat their own illnesses, either as individuals or as a family or similar small units. In other words, to alter the dial so that the dark 16% segment is narrowed while the 64% self-care segment is widened. There is bound to be a risk in this because, as many will point out, it means turning the clock back. "None practise physic nor professeth midwifery but charitably one neighbour helpeth another." Patients who need not have died will die and there must always be a conflict between the good of the individual and the good of the many. One dead child is a potent argument, far more potent than several children who might die if the medical services are overstretched.

I have the impression, which was to some extent borne out by the survey already mentioned, that patients who have a serious illness are more often aware of it than we suppose. Even an anxious or hypochondriacal patient will probably notice the difference within himself. The doctor, if he has his wits about him, will notice it too. It is like a change of key. This is some sort of safeguard, the other being that a delayed or faulty diagnosis is fortunately less likely to do harm than is generally supposed.

Home medicine can only be improved by education and I believe that this should be started at school. It must be acknowledged that the mother of the family always has been and still is the chief purveyor of medical care and to take this role from her is uneconomic and inefficient. Rather should she be trained to do the job well by sensible, practical instruction. This would best be done for girls at school. Theoretical medicine is confusing and not very helpful for lay people. To be able to draw a diagram of a streptococcus is of not the slightest value in treating a sore throat. To know the anatomy of the kidney is not important in the diagnosis of pyelitis. What is important is to know that a woman who has pain in the loin, does not feel well and keeps on running to the toilet almost certainly requires antibiotics. Practical observation of the Hippocratic type is what matters.

Teaching medicine to lay people is a double-edged weapon and when I look at some medical dictionaries and home-doctor books I feel like Wellington when he said, "I don't know what effect these men will have on the enemy but, by God, they terrify me". Fortunately good home-doctor books are just beginning to come on the market, although the older ones will no doubt remain in use, be reprinted and perpetuate fallacies for generations to come.

A 1958 edition of one medical dictionary in current use described treatment such as henbane for cystitis, steel-drops for anaemia and poppy-head fomentations for toothache. It mentioned electrical treatment for cancer and the section on pneumonia ended with an afterthought, "penicillin is often used now".

But a bigger danger than ignorance is sensationalism. Patients, of course, love this and approve of anything which makes their own illness more dramatic. A woman who has had a hysterectomy may say she was "four hours on the table and had everything taken away", and of course this is a good reason for her not doing the housework six months after the operation. Until recently the media, especially television, were guilty in this respect but it is good to see that programmes are becoming more enlightened. Television could be a potent weapon in teaching practical, sensible home medicine. Here is an example of almost incredible stupidity, in advertising, with no doubt the best of intentions.

Case 41 A married woman of 42 took part in a Cancer Fund Lottery. On the back of her ticket was printed "Unusual

> bladder symptoms indicate cancer". Since she was having one of her usual attacks of cystitis at the time she came to the surgery in a state of panic. The doctor found it difficult to convince her she had not got cancer.

Even lottery tickets could help if the advice they give is sensible, but I repeat that the chief source of education should be home medicine taught to girls at school from an early age as part of the curriculum. With examinations! This is only one way of escaping the horns of the dilemma. It has the advantage that it is more satisfying to be self-reliant and this is a philosophy of life which applies to many things apart from medicine.

To summarise I will quote the conclusions from the survey published in the Journal of the Royal College of General Practitioners.

> "It is suggested that home medical care plays an essential role in the structure of medical care as a whole and is still responsible for the majority of advice and treatment. It is a neglected subject because it is often supposed to be undesirable in a free and comprehensive health service".
>
> "There is no indication however that it will become obsolete in the forseeable future, nor any proof that this would be a desirable trend; in fact it may be an important part of family and community life. A plea is made for sensible and efficient training in home medical care, perhaps at school level, and further investigation into ways in which it might be extended to take away some of the burden of the National Health Service."

This applies not only to Britain but to any country in the world. A cynic, reading this, may remark, "What he is really saying is that doctors are becoming obsolete". This would be unjust because to me the medicine practised by doctors is by far the most important part of medical care but should, as far as possible, be applied only to illnesses where a doctor is needed. Medicine becomes more complicated day by day but illness remains the same. It is no coincidence that for centuries most illness has been treated by remedies called Simples and we should continue to use simple diagnosis and treatment for everything except the complex. "For the patient the least is best." This, of course, is a "simplification" of the problem because it leaves out the whole question of screening for hidden disease. Screening has its fanatical supporters and its equally fanatical opponents. For the patients, it is an unnatural process because they are seeking something they do not want, that is to say a disease. If some fault is found which in the opinion of the doctor requires treatment, such as symptomless hypertension or diabetes, the patient may not be enthusiastic about taking tablets for the rest of his life.

2.212 *It is only when diseases have established themselves, not while they are doing so, that the patient is ready to submit to treatment.*

It could be argued that the patient who is willing to be screened is seeking and finding reassurance. However the propaganda which persuades him to come may be the very thing which makes it necessary for him to have reassurance. Also most screening processes are repetitive. An annual medical examination suggests to the patient that he is all right for another year, a cervical smear test for another one to five years according to the report. My own feeling is that screening tests are of benefit to very few patients, harmful to quite a number in that faults are found which are unimportant or untreatable, neutral for the rest. I consider it unethical to bring too much pressure to bear on a patient unless the screening process is of proven benefit, such as ante-natal care. Time may prove me wrong.

7

The Art and the Conduct of the Doctor

2.311 *A doctor should look healthy and be of the correct weight, because ordinary folk think that a doctor who looks unfit cannot take care of others. He must be clean, well dressed and sweet-smelling. His reputation is enhanced if he is quiet in manner and known to lead a regular life. He must be a gentleman, grave and kind to all. Ostentation is despised, even though it may be useful.*

This is the traditional picture of a doctor. The matter of dress is important. Although the days of the frock coat, top hat and gold watch in the waist-coast pocket are long gone, most patients expect a doctor to look like a doctor. This means he should wear a suit although this need not be dark and sombre. In the country gumboots and other necessary impedimenta are acceptable but the doctor is expected to wear a tie. In hospital it is a sign of superiority not to wear a white coat. However, if it is worn it is a badge of office and should be clean and the clothes beneath it should be suitable.

Sadly it is nowadays sometimes difficult to tell a doctor from a hospital porter unless there is a stethoscope hanging from his pocket. It is commonplace to see hospital doctors with open-neck shirts and even wearing shorts under a white coat. Women doctors are as bad. The patients do not like this. I have sometimes visited a patient in hospital and asked if the doctor has been to see them only to receive in reply, "I don't know", because they genuinely did not know if the individual who came to see them was a doctor. It is also an insult to the nurses who are invariably correctly and neatly dressed. Hippocrates would not have permitted such doctors to sit and listen to him under his plane tree. Fortunately they are only a minority.

1.327 *You should not, in order to gain patients, use luxurious headgear and elaborate perfumes. Being too unconventional in dress will give you a bad reputation but a little unorthodoxy is in good taste. Yet I do not forbid you to please the patient by your appearance because this is not unworthy of a doctor's dignity.*

A doctor should never be overdressed but he should dress to advantage, because this is all part of Balint's "the drug doctor". An attractive woman doctor should use her attractiveness therapeutically but she should not be over- or under-dressed because, as already stated, the role of a mother, sister or wife goes with being a doctor: that of a mistress does not. Hippocrates does not object to a "little unorthodoxy" and patients like their doctors to be a bit of a character. The giants of old used to carry this to excess and I have seen a surgeon arrive to operate in the full dress uniform of an admiral. I also knew a physician who did his ward round in a long black cloak carrying a silver headed cane, which he would not release for a moment. This meant it was impossible for him to use a stethoscope, which was perhaps an advantage to all concerned. Few of us would aspire to such heights, but a rose in the buttonhole is pleasing and when I am a little older I think I will buy a gold Hunter watch. Looking at it is quite a performance and so much more relaxing than the nervous glance at the wrist watch. It makes time a thing of leisured importance.

There is much greater scope for country doctors, who may wear deer-stalker hats adorned with trout flies. A doctor I knew occasionally did his rounds on horseback, which was quite a practicable proposition for local calls. Another did winter visits on skis when the snow was deep but this was just to give him practice for his holiday in Switzerland. The doctor's car is, of course, an extension of his dress and if you want a quick assessment of his personality it may be helpful to look at the car first and the man second.

2.291 *The doctor must have at his command a certain ready wit, because a dour manner repels both the healthy and the sick. He must also keep a tight rein over himself, not exposing his deepest thoughts or gossiping with laymen, but saying only what is absolutely necessary. He should do nothing with fuss or show. This behaviour should be a matter of policy, otherwise he will fail when the need arises.*

The last sentence is a paraphrase of a difficult passage. I think Hippocrates means a doctor should train himself to behave in a certain manner even if his mood does not coincide with his actions. He should not show gloom, anger or boredom and he should refrain from talking about his own feelings and problems in the presence of a patient. If a doctor looks tired or is obviously busy most patients will be sympathetic. If he says "I was called out of bed twice last night" or "I'm going to miss my lunch today" his remark will fall flat and the patients' sympathy is diminished because they think he is complaining or even being hostile. After all it is not their fault if the doctor was called out at night.

A "certain ready wit" is extremely important and a doctor who has little sense of humour or cannot make his patients laugh is in a very difficult position. Laughter may be the only escape route from an intolerable position and the shared laughter with colleagues at coffee time is highly therapeutic for the doctor. It is a mistake to think that laughter and compassion are opposed to each other. Many doctors make outrageous jokes about matters which give them most concern. If the patients could hear they would be deeply shocked but there is no reason why they should be. It is, however, wise not to put humorous remarks in writing because, strangely enough, a patient or his representative has legal access to all case notes and the wittiest remark is often not very funny in open court.

Case 42 A young doctor in a maternity unit was called to a mother who gave birth to her baby prematurely in the toilet. In his letter to the patient's general practitioner he wrote "the baby was born in the lavatory pan but was fortunately able to swim". The secretary left this letter on a pile of others on a desk to await the doctor's signature and it was read by the hospital matron who passed it to the superintendent for action. The doctor was hard put to explain that this was a joke between professionals which had nothing to do with the seriousness of the event.

As far as the patients are concerned humour is one of the best therapeutic weapons, provided the doctor laughs with them and not at them. Most patients love gentle teasing but cannot tolerate sarcasm or scorn. The doctor must know when to laugh and when not to laugh. Quite often a patient will say, "I didn't come before because I was afraid you would laugh at me". He is deeply grateful because the doctor has listened seriously to something which appears trivial to everyone except himself.

Occasionally when a doctor makes a joke he will notice the expression on the patient's face becoming frozen. This is awkward and he will have to bluff his way out of it. It can sometimes be useful because he may have put his finger on a tender spot which can be explored tactfully at a later interview.

2.311 *He must make use of his liberty of action and should not be repetitious. In appearance he should be serious but not harsh, for harshness indicates arrogance and unkindness, while a man who does not control his laughter and excessive gaiety is vulgar and vulgarity must be avoided at all costs. He must be fair in all his social relationships. There is a close intimacy between the doctor and the patient. Patients in fact put themselves into the hands of their doctor and every day he meets women and girls with their precious possessions. Towards all these self control must be used. Such then should be the physician in body and mind.*

The matter of sexual feelings between doctor and patient has already been discussed. In case the reader thinks this is the beginning of the path to permissiveness he should study again these words of Hippocrates, and also the following extract from the General Medical Council's booklet "Professional Conduct and Discipline".

> "Patients grant doctors privileged access to their homes and confidences and some patients are liable to become emotionally dependent upon their doctors. Good medical practice depends upon the maintenance of trust between doctors and patients and their families and the understanding by both that proper professional relationships will be strictly observed. In this situation doctors must exercise great care and discretion in order not to damage this crucial relationship. Any action by a doctor which breaches this trust may raise the question of serious professional misconduct."

If I were to rewrite this excellent summary in slightly archaic style it could be passed off as part of the Hippocratic Collection. The booklet later explains that a doctor would be breaking his trust if he entered "into an emotional or sexual relationship with the patient (or with a member of a patient's family) which disrupts that patient's family life or otherwise damages, or causes distress to, the patient or his or her family".

Notice the order of the words "emotional or sexual". The general public likes to equate misconduct with sex but as much damage is done by emotional relationships which are relatively asexual. A doctor who displaces a relative, or friend for that matter, in the affections of a patient is on dangerous ground, and this may be in his role of father, son or what you will.

Case 43 A young doctor showed great kindness to an elderly lady who lived alone and visited her regularly for a chat. He was clearly playing the role of a son and her own children, who scarcely ever saw her, took exception to this. When she died she left the doctor a small gift in her will. This was handed over reluctantly. If she had left him a large sum of money there would have been a court case and the doctor would have been in the embarrassing position of proving he had not "exerted undue influence" over the old lady.

Regular social visits can be hazardous even when there is no question of a sexual relationship and the usual cause of trouble is guilt on the part of neglectful relatives. This should not deter the doctor if he thinks the patient is benefiting from it. The situation is explosive if there are remotely possible sexual aspects and the doctor should then insist on attendance at the surgery. Here he is relatively safe because, even if he is not chaperoned, his consulting room is within "screaming distance" of a receptionist. To see a patient at the surgery out of hours is folly yet one quite often reads of this in newspapers.

1.319 *I urge you not to be too unkind but to consider carefully your patient's superabundance or means. Sometimes give your services for nothing.*

This suggestion dates back to the old days where it was normal practice for a doctor to give his services free to the poor. In doing so he was "robbing the rich". This is now done officially by taxation so that most poor people have free medical services anyway. In backward countries it is a different story and extortion of the poor and ignorant is unforgivable. In one country it costs several months' wages to buy an injection of penicillin for a child with bilharzia, which is anyway not sensitive to penicillin.

I like to consider this passage in a human as well as a financial sense. Many patients lack "superabundance or means" in intelligence or education and the doctor should give his services for nothing, that is to say with no expectation of gratitude or appreciation. It is tempting to be annoyed by a patient who does not switch off the television, who talks to a relative while the doctor is examining him, or who does not say thank you. The doctor should "not be too unkind" in this sort of situation.

1.317 *For if you begin by discussing fees you will suggest to your patient that you will desert him if no agreement is reached or fail to give him immediate relief.*

Doctors nowadays rarely have to ask for money directly, this being left to a secretary or the tax man. There is argument as to whether financial transactions between doctor and patient are a good thing. It increases the value of what the doctor does but if handled tactlessly may upset the patient. If may also upset the doctor if he does not get his money. I heard of an old doctor who used to insist on collecting a half-crown piece from the mantelpiece before he would examine the patient, while his wife insisted on his handing over the half-crowns when he came home from his round and checked his visiting list to make sure none were missing.

1.323 *It is not against etiquette for a doctor who is in the dark through inexperience to call in others so, by consultation, he may learn the truth of the case. Doctors who meet in consultation must never quarrel or belittle each other. To be jealous is a sign of weakness and more suitable to the market place than to medicine. No matter how much help you have you can never have enough.*

Probably nothing lowers the prestige of doctors more than disagreement amongst themselves. If a doctor complains about a colleague or grumbles about his lot he will get no respect from the patient. It is likely to reflect back on himself or, if the patient is a gossip, find its way by devious means to the colleague who will resent it. Sometimes family doctors complain about the hospital or hospital doctors drop remarks about the patient's own doctor. A remark such as "It's a pity your doctor didn't send you up sooner" may destroy in a few seconds a longstanding mutual trust. Of course criticism is sometimes justified but hospital doctors are less critical if they have done a little general practice themselves. They will understand the waywardness of physical signs and the emotional pressures from relatives which barely infiltrate the hospital. It is difficult for a doctor to apply sound clinical judgement when an old grannie is muttering, "It's his appendix, you know", over his shoulder. He may send the child into hospital to be on the safe side or not send the child in through pique. Either way the hospital doctor may get a poor impression of him. This used to apply particularly to midwifery cases in the days when domiciliary deliveries were common. Officious relatives or neighbours used to say, "Hasn't the baby come yet?" every time the doctor put his head through the door, until he doubted his own judgement.

Consultation between doctors is essential and a doctor who works in isolation is likely to degenerate both in technical knowledge and attitude. Some are natural loners and many excellent country doctors see little of their colleagues, relying on support from their family or the patients themselves. In hospital it may work the other way round, there being inadequate isolation. This can be just as harmful.

It is important to remember that consultation is a two-way process and not only a handing over of knowledge by the senior to the junior, which is of limited value to either and probably boring. The senior should both learn and sharpen his wits.

1.299 *I will keep secret anything I shall see or hear in the course of my professional duties and in everyday life which should not be told to other people.*

Secrecy is a problem because a doctor must discuss his patient's affairs with his colleagues for his own and his patient's benefit. But who are his colleagues? Are they other doctors? Are they nurses and health visitors who work with him? Are they people with no special medical training such as social workers, receptionists, secretaries, clergy or indeed anyone who has an interest in the patient's welfare? I think Hippocrates would advise the doctor to use his judgement in each case. Some matters are so personal and upsetting for the patient that they should not be discussed with anyone or even recorded in the notes, which is a form of remote consultation. The doctor should consider the patient's wishes and what benefit he will obtain. He will not usually need to ask permission for disclosure of information to his colleagues or staff. After all the typist will probably know. But he should think carefully before talking to people outside his own practice or hospital unit, for example with clergy or social workers. This is partly a matter of personalities and the doctor will feel freer with, say, a social worker attached to his practice or unit, whom he knows, than a voice over the 'phone.

The doctor should also be careful about filling in forms for insurance companies or for applications for jobs. Signed permission by the patient is not an ethical carte blanche. The doctor's wife is another special case. "Pillow conversation" may be necessary for the doctor's peace of mind and a good night's sleep but he must be careful not to mention names of people known to his family except in a general sense.

There are gossips in all departments of life and God protect the patient from a gossiping doctor! The doctor will eventually need a barrister as well as God.

1.299 *I will not procure abortion in a woman.*

This is a statement with no ifs or buts. It must give pause for thought. One could say the ifs or buts have evolved since Hippocrates' time – such as safety of the operation, methods of identifying an abnormal foetus, and the social catastrophe of the population explosion. Nonetheless Hippocrates holds that abortion is wrong. Scientifically speaking the person exists from the moment of conception because the genes carry the blueprint of his future and to kill the blueprint is to kill a personality. A destroyed foetus is forever a might-have-been and the mother may be aware of this for the rest of her life. As T. S. Eliot put it:

> "What might have been is an abstraction . . .
> Footfalls echo in the memory
> Down the passage we did not take
> Towards the door we never opened. . . ."

There is no scientific justification for insisting on termination before the twelfth week. It is just that we feel more squeamish as the foetus gets larger and we would certainly not agree with the Greek custom of exposing newborn infants. This was considered socially justifiable in Hippocrates' time but was not within the province of a doctor.

Here we have another dilemma, not an enjoyable one. There

are two ways of escape. The first is to accept that abortion is evil but failure to abort may be a greater evil. In other words every termination should be accepted as an individual moral problem and not as a foregone conclusion. The second is to put the matter outside the jurisdiction of doctors, who express their opinion but are not responsible for decision or action. This lies between the patient and the State, which represents a cultural attitude. The big arguments against this is that it would lead to "committee decisions" which tend to be long winded and less responsible than a personal decision by someone who knows the patient. And who is better for this than a family doctor? The debate continues.

1.299 *I will keep my personal life and my word pure and upright.*

The two, of course, are inseparable. Although a doctor must be to some extent an actor, it is difficult to sustain a part indefinitely. If there is something wrong with his life it will, in time, affect his work and his relationship with patients, either by slow infiltration or sudden explosion. I will not try to define the word "wrong". The doctor will make his own judgement. It includes such qualities as unkindness, dishonesty with himself or others and sexual deception. One of course hears tales of learned and respected physicians who lead a double life and it is interesting that when Robert Louis Stevenson wrote the story of Jekyll and Hyde he made Jekyll a doctor. As everyone knows, Hyde could not be kept under control and this, in a less dramatic way, will happen to most doctors who play that particular game.

Less spectacular but also important is the minor cheating which goes on in the medical profession. I can remember as a trainee general practitioner many years ago one of my less salutary tasks was to empty some twenty bottles of urine down the drain after each antenatal clinic. The specimens were never tested but the patients were in trouble if they failed to bring their bottle. This was deception.

I still sometimes have to pretend I can see the retina with an ophthalmoscope, even using a modern instrument – the older type appeared to be designed to show only a reflection from the nearest window. It is wiser to do this than to tell the patient "I cannot see anything". I also once deceived an asthmatic patient by giving an injection of water when I had forgotten to bring adrenalin. It worked well. These minor deceptions are necessary to cover up poor organisation. It is not, however, "upright" behaviour, although from the patient's point of view it is often the correct thing to do.

1.299 *I will not administer harmful substances to anyone if asked to do so, nor will I suggest such an action.*

This is another definite statement. Hippocrates opposed euthanasia and would, I think, do so equally strongly today. If a doctor breaks his pledge in this matter there is no going back. It is a progressive step with ever widening indications for ending life, and those whom he would not wish to die today he may destroy without much thought tomorrow. Starting with terminal illness, senility and congenital abnormalities he may travel the long path to social undesirability from any cause whatsoever. As we well know this can mean political views, race, colour, stupidity, maladjustment and crime to the final dictum that "Anyone I do not think should live has no right to". This is no longer a medical matter, but the worst of those Nazi doctors who collaborated with mass murder probably began by making some slightly questionable clinical decision. As Hamlet said of a different matter, each act or abstinence "shall lend a kind of easiness to the next . . . : the next more easy; For use almost can change the stamp of nature".

Hippocrates would stand firm on this, but like all doctors he would not have withheld large doses of drugs from those dying in distress nor would he treat energetically those in whom death is of secondary importance. The reader may say that the last statement bring us back to square one. It is, however, a question of the intention rather than the act and it is worth repeating Arthur Hugh Clough's version of the sixth commandment:

> "Thou shalt not kill; but need'st not strive
> Officiously to keep alive."

A doctor who makes a clinical decision not to give treatment to a doomed person at either extreme of life should make his intention clear to the nursing staff, who may have developed fondness even for an inanimate patient. He should use his judgement with relatives. Some benefit from being consulted, others fear even helping with a decision of this sort and are permanently loaded with guilt.

1.299 *I will undertake no act which I am inadequately trained to perform but will leave it to those who are expert.*

Being qualified as a doctor does not mean being qualified to undertake all work done by all doctors. Medical qualification is becoming more and more meaningless. For example most "bachelors of chirurgery" are quite incapable of undertaking the simplest of operations. Similarly a professor of surgery would be a menace as a family doctor, although he might not have the insight to realise this. A doctor has a right to refuse to do anything he cannot do reasonably well but should consider whether it is up to him to learn. The legal and moral aspects of this are at present confused.

General medical qualifications and general medical training are probably still valid because this gives an insight into medicine as a whole and in a crisis a poor craftsman is better than none at all.

Case 44 A family doctor was called by a midwife at 2 a.m. to a home confinement. The mother was near full dilatation and the midwife thought the baby was presenting as a breech. On his way in the car the sleepy doctor was trying to remember all he could about breech deliveries, not having witnessed one for about ten years. He visualised a passage in a textbook which said, "Do nothing until the buttocks are delivered then let them hang down". He arrived just as the breech was showing but after a few minutes it became clear that it was not advancing. He now saw, again as if written in a textbook, the words "Never pull on the breech". Using gas and air analgesia only he did a vaginal examination and managed to pull both legs down. He then felt both arms extended alongside the head and by bending these at the elbow – again from memory – and twisting the baby to and fro he was finally able to pull the arms down and deliver the after coming head with forceps. In spite of this amateurish treatment the baby was born in good conditions except she developed a sternomastoid tumor due to muscle damage. The doctor got back to bed at 4.30 a.m. but did not sleep the rest of the night. It is of great interest that nine years later the child developed Perthe's disease of the hip. Was there a connection?

These last excerpts have been taken from the Hippocratic Oath which is recorded in full at the end of the book.

1.299 *If I carry out this oath I hope to gain a good reputation as a doctor and a person. If I fail to carry it out I will expect to get what I deserve.*

8

The Art and Creative Diagnosis

2.7 *I think it an excellent thing for a doctor to practise forecasting. For if by listening at the bedside he can find out about the past, the present and the future, then fill in the gaps for himself, he will be more believed and trusted.*

What did Hippocrates mean by "filling in the gaps"? It could imply no more than asking routine questions to supplement the patient's story, about such matters as bowel and bladder function, which make a "complete history". These are a bore for the junior hospital doctor and are usually omitted by the family doctor. Or it could refer to more searching relevant questions designed to track down a particular disease. The wording is tantalising and almost smacks of dishonesty. "Filling in the gaps for *himself*". For me it leads towards a way of thinking which Hippocrates did not mention directly but about which he would, as I hope to show, have been aware.

This thinking process is associated today with what is called Gestalt psychology. *Gestalt* is the German for "form" or "shape" and the idea is that perception is concerned with patterns and relationships rather than individual stimuli. Thus if you look for a moment at fifty dots arranged in a circle you will see the circle not the fifty dots. You will probably be unaware that the circle is made of dots. Similarly if you are shown a triangle of which a small section is missing you will see a complete triangle. This is called the Law of Closure, which implies that the mind "fills in the gaps" where possible to make a complete picture. In other words perception is never a simple photographic-type recording but a fitting of sensations into a pattern which is anticipated or wished for.

The fundamentalists of the Behaviourist school tried to base perception on the idea of simple reflex arcs. It was thought that Pavlov's dogs salivated when they smelled their dinners because of an automatic electrical system which had nothing to do with their feelings about the dinner. They *had* to salivate and the fact that they looked forward with pleasurable anticipation to a meal was a side-issue. By a process of conditioning, other reflex arcs could be created so that the dog could be taught to salivate at the sound of a bell. It was thought that these arcs were actual electric circuits in the brain and perception was a process similar to switching on a light or dialling a 'phone number. If the arcs were intentionally confused the wires would become crossed and the dog would become neurotic, either barking in frustration or giving up and becoming immobile. This was the basis of mental illness, the forerunner of an anxiety state on the one hand and a depressive illness on the other.

Although Pavlov's theories were a great advance in psychology they can be easily disproved, at any rate in their strict anatomical aspect. When a man, or a dog, looks at an object his eyes are continually flickering so he must be activating thousands of arcs. His perception therefore cannot be a simple electrical procedure. It can only be explained by perception of a pattern or relationship. If in fact a visual image is fixed, and the only way to do this is to paint a picture on a contact lens, perception becomes distorted and the image fades and partially disappears. A simple arc cannot take constant stimulation.

The most telling disproof of a mechanistic form of perception lies in the famous experiments of Lashley. He went to the great trouble of teaching mice to find their way through a maze, then the even greater trouble of removing small sections of their cerebral cortex, 5% at a time. He found this made remarkably little difference to their ability to follow the maze, whichever part of the cortex was excised. There was a gradual falling off of competence as larger portions were removed but even a mouse with one half of his total cortex destroyed coped reasonably well. The point was that the competence of the mouse depended on the quantity not the site of the brain tissue removed and this makes nonsense of a theory of perception based on fixed electric circuits.

To a psychologist all this is elementary and obvious but to the general reader it may not be. To take another example, while you are reading this book you are not perceiving each letter or each word as something individual, unless you happen to be an illiterate who is just beginning to learn the great art of reading. You see words in groups and, if you are a very rapid reader, you may see lines in groups. The process is as much intelligent guess-work as actually seeing. For this reason I could slip in misprints galore and most of them would pass unnoticed, because you would automatically fit them into a pattern. Proof-readers know all about this. They have to obliterate the pattern and the sense of what they are reading and concentrate on individual words. This is very difficult to do. I once wrote an article on the treatment of bedwetting with a buzzer and it was only in the third reading that someone noticed that instead of "electric buzzer" the typist had, to her shame, put "electric bugger" as a cure for enuresis.

If this general theory of Gestalt perception were incorrect, artists would be out of work because the only valid art would be the photograph. As it is, a skilful artist can draw a few lines on a piece of paper and rely on the viewer to create the rest. He makes his money because the viewer enjoys creating his own pictures, whereas he would be bored stiff if given a photograph album to look at. Thus perception is always a creative process and the person can create what he expects, what he wants or, if he is mentally ill, what he dreads. This is the basis of the famous Rorschach Inkspot Test, where patients create fantasies out of shapes, a game that has been played since the beginning of mankind. The Greeks saw constellations in the pattern of the stars, Cassiopoea on her couch, the great Orion striding through the heavens with Sirius the dogstar at his heels. Shakespeare knew all about it. Witness this speech by Mark Antony in the moment of bitterness when he knew Cleopatra had betrayed him:

> "Sometimes we see a cloud that's dragonish;
> A vapour sometime like a bear or lion,
> A tower'd citadel, a pendant rock,
> A forked mountain, or blue promontory
> With trees upon 't, that nod unto the world
> And mock our eyes with air: thou hast seen those signs;
> They are black vesper's pageants."

Because perception is creative everyone sees things in different ways and the same person sees the same object in different ways at different times. The phenomenon of alternating figures is well known. If you look at the diagram below you will see either a goblet or two faces and will be able consciously to flash from one to the other.

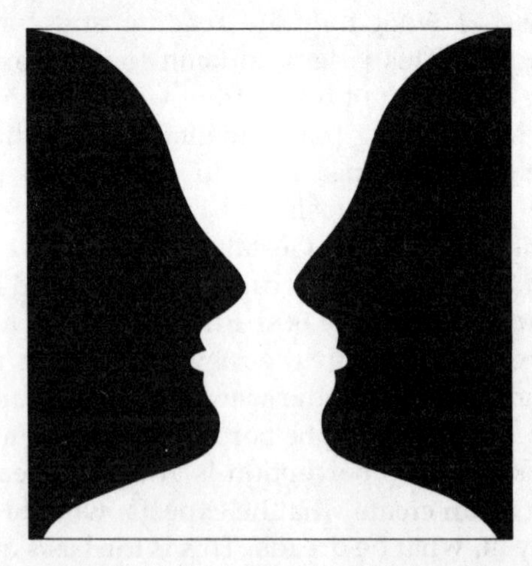

What has this to do with medicine and Hippocrates? A lot. If we believe that perception is a creative process and the perceiver selects a few of the mass of stimuli presented to him and uses his imagination to create a picture, then we can say the same about clinical diagnosis. For diagnosis is but an extended form of perception and we even use the expression "clinical picture" as if we were artists rather than doctors.

1.313 *We must conceive of our nature being stirred and receiving sensations by compulsion from a great number of things: and the intellect, taking over from nature, the impression, leads us afterwards to the truth.*

How do we make this picture? We receive a number of stimuli from our patient. Most important perhaps are the auditory stimuli or history, the greater part of which we probably discard as irrelevant but fill in the gaps either by direct questioning, using our imagination, or both. Questions may be designed to get the answers we expect. At the same time we receive non-verbal messages, the facial play, the tightly clenched hands, the sweat on the brow, the way the patient sits. As Richard Asher said, a patient's anxiety can be measured by the distance of his sacrum to the back of the chair. By now the picture is forming, so we carry out a physical examination and our eyes, hands and ears fill in more gaps or even finds gaps we did not expect. All the while these masses of stimuli are being mixed and sorted by a kind of Identikit method and the various pictures we paint are compared with other pictures we have seen or read about in the past. At last by laborious work or a swift stroke of the brush we have what we believe to be the true picture and say to ourselves, "Ah, thyrotoxicosis!" or whatever it is, just as a viewer in an art gallery will look at a picture and say, "Ah, Rembrandt". We say "thyrotoxicosis" because we have seen similar pictures with the same name before and this matches. An experienced doctor who has, as it were, spent years walking art galleries will recognise the picture by its style and may even have made the diagnosis at a glance. For him history and examination is for confirmation only, as it were framing the picture rather than painting it. It may even be done out of politeness to the patient, the doctor having to demonstrate that he finds the picture worth more than a casual glance.

The less experienced doctor will come to a diagnosis step by step by enumerating specific points. He builds up his picture piece-meal rather like an amateur painter who buys the sort of painting kit where you fill in squares in different colours by numbers. The end result is a reasonable reproduction and may look well on the sitting-room wall provided it is not examined too closely. It will not be an inspired work and the inexperienced doctor will marvel at or doubt the clinical acumen of his senior. He may even be annoyed because he has struggled to learn, for example, the fifteen features of thyrotoxicosis but these have not been fused into a pattern which gives an instant diagnosis.

1.329 *Experience is useful, the learning of other people's opinions far less so.*

An example will be given of this. In a training session an actor was coached in the role of an elderly man with myxoedema. He was presented to two doctors in front of an audience, one a top-class trainee in general practice, the other an experienced and highly thought of trainer. The trainee went through a series of selective questions-and-answers based on the knowledge he possessed from previous teaching and by a process of deduction decided the patient was suffering from depression and, because time was limited, arranged a further appointment to unravel the causes of this and decide on treatment.

The trainer looked at the patient as he came in, noted he was wearing an overcoat although the weather was warm, noted his slow responses and in a flash had painted a picture of myxoedema. He asked a single question, "You seem to feel the cold a lot, don't you, Mr. Smith?" The answer gave the diagnosis and the rest of the interview was spent in touching up the picture. As has been said the trainee was an outstanding doctor but in this instance he failed to pick up non-verbal clues because he was keen to make a diagnosis by asking the right questions. The audience commented that there was less "contact" with the trainee than with the trainer. The trainer actually touched the patient on several occasions, for example, helping him off with his coat. This made the patient more satisfied with the interview because he had undergone grooming behaviour, as Desmond

Morris would describe it. Also he realised the trainer had painted an accurate picture while the trainee was fiddling about with his brushes, putting a dab here and a dab there. Naturally the sitter appreciates a good portrait of himself. The type of situation can be repeated over and over again with similar results but the less experienced doctor can console himself that in ten years' time it will be he who knows the answer "intuitively", that is to say he has developed a style of his own which consists of contact with the patient as well as awareness of the disease.

A psychologist reading this will not be impressed. He will say, "All you have done is to put in rather high flown language what is obvious. We have used special techniques for examining such matters for years. You have described something and have not, in truth, attempted to interpret it. In fact by talking about artists and paintings you have confused the issue and made it less valid." This comment I challenge. Without decrying the work of experimental psychologists – and I count myself as one in that I hold a degree in the subject – I consider they often err by taking emotion and symbolic thought out of their work. In trying to increase accuracy by being objective they often become less accurate because what they are measuring is non-existent or at least unimportant. Taking the bust measurement of the Venus de Milo does nothing to enhance her beauty, but this is the kind of situation the psychologist finds himself in. He must measure, and if there is nothing worth measuring, he must think of something. It is for this reason too that most books on experimental psychology "for the general reader" are heavy going. One of the dicta of Gestalt psychology is that the sum is greater than the parts, so the study of the parts is often of slight value as well as being terribly boring.

Having written these words I should retract them at once because Hippocrates would not have altogether agreed with me. In one of the dialogues Plato describes a discussion between Socrates and Phaedrus in which Socrates makes a long winded statement which I have paraphrased:

I xxxiii. "Observe what both Hippocrates and correct argument mean by the study of nature. First decide if the matter is simple or complex. If it is simple we must ask ourselves how it acts and upon what. If it is complex we must divide it into simple components and deal with each in the same way."

Sabin, of polio vaccine fame, recently made a similar statement on television. He said, "Complex questions must be split into small questions and these must be answered individually. This is sheer drudgery, but eventually all these little bits will form a pattern and the main question is answered."

The dilemma can be solved by saying that it is justifiable to study a part provided you remember it is a part. It is all too easy to become so specialised that a view of the whole is lost. A surgeon is a specialist who may have little insight into his patient's problem unless he considers himself "a physician who operates". He may even become a super-specialist and consider his own speciality, say the brain or the heart, in isolation. He will lose much as a doctor if he does this although his technical skill is not in question.

In brief, anything which is taken to bits must be put together again, or as Hippocrates expressed it:

1.315 *For so I think the whole art has been set forth, by observing some part of the final end in each of many particulars and then combining all into a single whole.*

If we are to accept the Gestalt view in relation to clinical diagnosis we should try it out on some cases. I have chosen three; one simple, another less simple, and a third complex.

Case 45 A boy of nine was admitted to hospital with a doctor's letter on which was written "? Appendicitis". The house surgeon naturally approached the bed with this particular Identikit picture in his mind which, in fact, dates back to Hippocrates.

2.17 *A swelling of the abdomen which is hard and painful is worse if it extends all over the abdomen. Should it be on one side only it is more dangerous on the right.*

However, because his last patient with abdominal pain

had a streptococcal sore throat and mesenteric adenitis he had a second Identikit picture in reserve. Behind this there were many other pictures representing diseases which might have been relevant, from the common to the most obscure. The doctor decided to take the history from the mother and because he was in a hurry he did this in the form of a leading question: "I gather your son's been getting tummy pain. Tell me about it". The house surgeon was lucky. With a little prompting the mother told him the pain had started in the centre of the abdomen then moved over to the right. The child had vomited once and his bowels had not been open. The pattern was almost complete, so the house surgeon next examined the abdomen and found tenderness and guarding in the right iliae fossa. It all fitted in beautifully and the house surgeon, if he was visually minded, might actually have seen an image of an inflamed appendix. He made a few more routine remarks but his mind was already set on organising the theatre for an appendicectomy. He was probably entirely satisfied, but in fact his picture had not been very well painted because it failed to show important details. The child was petrified with fright. The mother was in a quandary because she did not know whether she should stay with him or go home to her other three children. However, the diagnosis served its purpose. The appendix was removed and everyone was happy, except perhaps the child and his mother who remembered their fears and doubts. The house surgeon probably never realised his picture was incomplete.

The next case was far more complicated. It was an unusual affair in which painting was important literally as well as the symbolic painting of a clinical picture.

Case 46 An actress was taking the part of Lucifer in a Miracle Play. For this role the exposed parts of her body had to be covered in silver paint so that, at a critical moment, she could simulate Lucifer, the morning star in his pride, falling into the sea. She attended the surgery, rather unromantically complaining of itching, which was so bad she had difficulty in getting through the performance without scratching. The Identikit of allergy to silver paint matched so well that the doctor failed to notice that the papular rash did not coincide with the area where the paint had been applied. It was like not noticing a gap in a triangle in a Gestalt experiment and applying the Law of Closure. He made Lucifer do without her silver paint and she used instead a steroid cream together with antihistamines by mouth. This had little effect apart from making her sleepy so a dermatologist was asked to see her. He at once diagnosed scabies, the picture fitting in with his past experience of that disease. The family doctor had not included an actress and a nasty infective condition in the same pattern but, as the dermatologist pointed out, Lucifer was just the person one would expect to catch scabies.

These two cases were relatively straightforward. The first was a familiar and clear cut clinical picture of appendicitis but the doctor was not sufficiently creative to extend the picture to fit the circumstances. The second was a false pattern built on two misconceptions – that an unfamiliar substance applied to the skin must be the cause of the irritation and that beautiful girls do not get scabies.

The third case is far more complex, being the life story of a psychiatric patient. It will be presented in three ways each with a different degree of creativeness. At the end the reader must decide which is nearest the truth, if indeed truth is a useful word in this context. The three interpretations are very different from each other and will require a conscious change of attitude on the part of the reader.

Case 51a J.C. was a case of chronic paranoid schizophrenia, presenting as acute delusional states in an introspective personality subject to fantasising. These episodes became increasingly more severe and were exacerbated by a change of domicile, leading to admission to a mental hospital. At this time J.C. identified himself with well known persons who were ego-symbols and there was also a strong marital–sexual content, in which ideas of bigamy were dominant. The disease ran a fluctuating course with reasonable insight being retained. After four years he absconded but was soon readmitted under Section to a second mental hospital. The disease became slowly progressive but he retained some insight with ability to relate to people and natural objects. He was allowed freedom of movement, being restrained only during relapses, but dementia gradually ensued and he died 23 years after admission, following a stroke.

Case 51b

John Clare, who is sometimes referred to as the "Northamptonshire peasant poet", was born on July 13th, 1793 in the tiny village of Helpstone, near Peterborough. He came from a poor family but because of the close ties in those days between the Big House and the tenants, he had access to the library of the Fitzwilliam family. He was thus able to spend part of his time reading and part wandering round the country observing nature.

He wrote poems about what he saw, the trees, the birds, the people in his village, with accuracy and in a style which can only be described as colloquial. His tragedy was that his poems suddenly became fashionable. He was "a charming rustic poet" overnight. The aristocracy took him up and he became the protégé of Lord Radstock and a rather silly lady called Mrs Emmerson. Just as quickly he was dropped. In 1827 his publisher Taylor, also the publisher of Keats, wrote, "The season has been a bad one for new books and I am afraid that the time has passed away in which poetry will answer." Clare continued to write reams of verse which no one wanted to read.

There were other tragedies. He had been in love with a girl called Mary Joyce but because he was socially inferior the engagement was broken off and he consoled himself with an illiterate girl called Patty. She became pregnant, so he had to marry her. His mind was split between the idyllic Mary and the mundane Patty until, later, he believed he was bigamously married to both.

The country he loved was an area of roughly three by three miles. It was the time of the Enclosure Act and he saw the familiar countryside being destroyed before his eyes, feeling probably much as people today who watch a housing estate being built on their favourite fields. He became impoverished and mentally ill, having attacks of what he called the Blue Devils. The Fitzwilliam family, ever kind, found him a free cottage four miles away in the village of Northborough but, so parochial were people in those days, that it was like emigrating to a foreign country. This contributed to his final breakdown. He had delusions, believing himself to be Byron,

Burns and other people he admired, and was at last admitted to High Beech Asylum at Epping. After four years he absconded and walked all the way to Peterborough, sleeping by the roadside and eating grass "which seemed to taste something like bread". Near Northborough he was met by Patty in a farm cart. But it was Mary he sought and the last entry in his remarkable diary "A Journey out of Essex" reads: "July 24th. 1841. Returned home out of Essex and found no Mary – her and her family are nothing to me now though she herself was once the dearest of all – and how can I forget". She had in fact died six years previously.

Clare was soon back in hospital, this time the Northampton County Asylum. Here he was treated with remarkable humanity, considering that at the time of his birth it had been customary to keep lunatics chained in straw and for the public to pay entrance fees to come and laugh at them. He was allowed to wander round the town and was encouraged to write poetry, which was preserved by the house steward W. F. Knight. Mental deterioration was gradual and he died following a stroke in 1864.

Case 51c (This should be read slowly, line by line.)

"I am – yet what I am, none cares or knows;
My friends forsake me like a memory lost;
I am the self-consumer of my woes –
They rise and vanish in oblivions host,
Like shadows in love's frenzied stifled throes
And yet I am, and live – like vapours tost

Into the nothingness of scorn and noise,
Into the living sea of waking dreams,
Where there is neither sense of life or joys,
But the vast shipwreck of my life's esteems;
Even the dearest that I love the best
Are strange – nay, rather, stranger than the rest.

I long for scenes where man has never trod
A place where woman never smiled or wept
There to abide with my Creator God,
And sleep as I in childhood sweetly slept,
Untroubling and untroubled where I lie
The grass below, above, the vaulted sky."

Three aspects of the same case, the last being the poem "I am" by John Clare himself, written during a period of insight while in a mental hospital. (This is one of several versions of the poem which have come down to us.)

The first history is something of a caricature of which any psychiatrist would be ashamed. It is arid and non-creative. The patient is almost anonymous and is mentioned as infrequently as possible. It is, in fact, an Identikit of paranoid schizophrenia which could be applied to many other similar cases. The patient, and incidentally the doctor, escape through the net. The aim is to establish a diagnosis. As so often happens in psychiatric illness more than one Identikit picture will fit and some students of John Clare believe him to have been manic-depressive. Others consider he suffered from pure paranoia, which was described by Kraepelin as "the insidious development of a permanent and unshakeable delusional system arising from internal causes which is accompanied by perfect preservation of clear and orderly thinking, willing and acting". If Clare were still alive the matter could no doubt be settled but it is not very important, although it is interesting to speculate on the effect Largactil would have had on his poetry.

The second history is a factual but imaginative summing up of Clare's life, leading to a diagnosis of paranoid schizophrenia. His mind was split between Patty and Mary, between peasant and poet, between working class and aristocracy, between Helpstone and Northborough. This split mind evolved into paranoia. We feel we know a lot about Clare and the passage from his "Journey out of Essex" increases the poignancy. The writer has created a pattern of what he thought about Clare and what he knew about paranoid schizophrenia. It is interesting and informative and for these reasons the reader will probably remember it.

The third history *is* John Clare. This is as creative a piece of writing as one could find anywhere. The word schizophrenia is not mentioned and does not have to be, because it is irrelevant. Yet there has never been a better description of depersonalisation, turning inwards, living in a twilight world with no feeling, estrangement from loved ones, longing for oblivion, for childhood, for death. Because it is poetry it means far more than a factual case history or a paragraph in a text book.

The language is largely symbolic and needs interpretation by the reader, from whom is demanded some poetic sensibility. If it is read repeatedly it gains in meaning, because creativeness is itself creative. The reader will understand a little about mental illness and even something about himself. He is advised, at this point, to turn back and read the poem again carefully.

All this may seem a far cry from the consulting room or hospital and we cannot really expect the doctor to write his notes in rhyming verse. But we should expect him, if he is a complete doctor, to have the ability to interpret illness in a creative (or, if you like, poetic) way.

Superficially this appears to be the "onion hypothesis" all over again. In fact it is almost the reverse. The writer of the first version starts with the word schizophrenia which he believes to be the centre of the onion and adds a few layers. The writer of the third version, John Clare himself, also starts at what he believes to be the centre, his own feelings. Only the writer of the second version is a traditional onionist, starting from the outside and stripping off layers.

Which is nearest the truth? This we have to decide for ourselves and our choice will depend much on our own personality. More of this later.

Hippocrates himself did not include poetry in his Collection, except for one couplet from Homer:

3.217 *As when the season of Spring arrives,*
Welcome to crumple-horned cattle.

One can scarcely imagine a less inspiring piece of verse and it was not very relevant to the subject he was discussing. Since, however, the Collection is basically a manual of practical medicine one would not expect poetry to play a part.

This does not mean that literature, and poetic drama in particular, was not important to Hippocrates in relation to his work. The opposite is probably true. He lived in an age when Dramatic Contests were almost a national sport, comparable to football today, and he was a close contemporary of Sophocles and Euripides, who probably rank in the top ten of playwrights since the world began. The Greeks had the extraordinary genius of developing scientific and poetic thought at one and the same time, and the two were closely linked.

The triple case history of the poet John Clare would not have seemed strange to Hippocrates because this represents the way the Greeks thought, a combination of scientific observation and poetic insight. Hippocrates himself comes to us across the centuries as a man of great sensibility as well as wisdom, and his so-called beside manner, that is to say his kindness and understanding, were in part a reflection of the literature being created at the time. I like to think of Euripides as his alter ego.

Literature was then, and still is, important to the Art of Medicine because it explores the aspirations of the human mind in the way that the present day psychologists fail to do. Freud attempted to understand the mind by narrowing it to concepts which are themselves narrow. He thus limited himself to a framework as bare as the hull of a sunken ship. A great writer sets himself no limits and therefore creates a more accurate and perceptive image. To read a good book, or play, is to see the ship in full sail and have a good idea what each member of the crew is up to.

Hippocrates had no Freud, or any other psychiatrist, to help him although some of his own writings anticipated Freud. This may have been in his favour because it allowed him a better understanding of his patients. He had Aeschylus, Sophocles and Euripides behind him, just as we have Shakespeare and Ibsen or, for that matter, Beethoven and Michelangelo.

This does not mean we should set up the creative approach to medicine as a rival either to the science of medicine or to what is commonly called psychology. It is part of a triad and a part that tends to be neglected in favour of the other two. This should not be so and those who find sensibility to the Arts important or essential to their practice of medicine should not be afraid to speak their minds.

Happily, the medical journals of today are beginning to support this approach which, apart from anything else, makes them much more readable. The British Medical Journal, for example, has several pages in each issue concerned with literature and creative writing while World Medicine fights a veritable crusade against what I call the illiteracy of modern medicine with the traditional weapons of common sense, wit and satire. This is very important because technical or jargon terms can only portray a part of the pattern of the patient and his illness.

To summarise this chapter, diagnosis like perception is a creative process. The doctor may think he is being objective but is using his imagination to create a picture. In simple illnesses, such as a sore throat, the creativeness will be slight unless the doctor wishes to extend the diagnosis to the family relationships of which the sore throat is a part. When faced with a difficult clinical problem or an illness in which the patient's personality is paramount the doctor must draw on all his resources. As well as his clinical knowledge and experience this includes sensibility of an artistic kind. Unless the doctor can combine the two he cannot make a complete diagnosis or be a complete doctor.

9

Learning and Teaching the Art

Hippocrates was renowned as a teacher and his seminars under the plane tree on the island of Cos have become a legend. It is disappointing that he says little about his teaching methods. One would give one's eyes to be able to go back in time and sit on the outskirts of the group in the shade of the tree and find out exactly what went on. It can only be presumed that the seminars were similar to the dialogues of Socrates in which ideas were bandied backwards and forwards, often coming more and more abstruse until they evaporated into nothing.

> ". . . and heard great argument
> About it and about: but evermore
> Came out by the same door as in I went."

Or maybe it was not like this. Hippocrates was such a practical man that he might have preferred to bring the conversation down to a more mundane level – the precise time to lance an abscess, the technique of setting fractures, the exact dilution of wine to be drunk when the body is heated. One can imagine him saying, "That's all very well but how can we apply this idea to the case of Philiscus who lives by the Wall?" There is a modern parallel to this.

Hippocrates is most famed as a teacher because of his concept of bedside teaching. This was probably his greatest contribution to medicine and has been handed down to the present day, although there have been dark ages of medicine when it has been in abeyance. In most universities in the 17th century a medical student could go through his entire training without seeing a patient. He was stuffed with background knowledge. The foreground did not matter. The university of Leiden was one of the few places where practical medicine was taught and students flocked to it from all over Europe.

Hippocrates was at times scathing about the standards of medicine of his day and the poor quality of the teaching:

2.263 *Medicine is the most distinguished of all the arts but it is by now the least thought of because of the ignorance of those who practise it and the casual way people judge such practitioners.*

This really was a condemnation of the medical profession and possibly Hippocrates had in mind the wicked Cnidians, also the many non-professionals who impersonated doctors but kept well out of their way if they got into difficulties.

1.321 *For quacks do not attempt treatment when they see an alarming condition and avoid calling in other physicians because they wickedly hate help.*

Today we can be more optimistic. In popularity opinion polls doctors invariably come near the top just as politicians usually come near the bottom. Do doctors deserve this? At least they are there to help people and are seen to be helping them, while politicians are considered to be obstructive and two-faced, more interested in policies and taxes than people. This is unfair, but anything that goes wrong is thought to be their fault and the excuses they give on television are often feeble in the extreme. More important they have little personal contact with the people except for hasty door-to-door visiting at election times and patting babies on the head on charity occasions. It is probably no coincidence that M.P.s in Britain hold what they call "surgeries" for their constituents but, from what I hear, these bear little resemblance to a doctor's surgery because all too often they have nothing to offer apart from promises they know they cannot keep. The doctor on the other hand is reasonably accessible, in spite of the protectiveness of his receptionist and delays in the hospital service. He also has something to give. Most patients leave the surgery clutching a prescription, often symbolic, while no constituent leaves his M.P.s surgery clutching the deeds to a new house. But doctors should not be too complacent. Nurses are usually ahead of them in the popularity polls, because they are, on the whole, kinder and have closer personal contact with the patient.

Doctors are lucky because they have a good image. In plays, books and serials they are nearly always the heroes, and even if they turn out to be villains they are, like Dr Crippen, at least interesting villains. So the "casual way people judge practitioners" works on the whole to their advantage. Ignorance and even rudeness are glossed over but it will not necessarily remain so, and this brings us to the importance of teaching good medicine and good behaviour to medical students and for doctors to continue to develop these after they have qualified.

2.263 *A person who has true knowledge of medicine must have natural ability, teaching, a suitable place to learn, education from childhood, hard work and time.*

It is interesting that Hippocrates should state that education starts from childhood. He might have added that it finishes on the day the doctor retires from work.

Recently there have been complaints that the education c. doctors from childhood makes them purveyors of so-called middle-class morality. Either they come from a middle-class background or have middle-class ideas grafted onto them during their schooling. They do not thus represent the ordinary person. There is some truth in this but much water will flow under the bridge before the general public will want it otherwise. Most patients share with Hippocrates the conception of what a doctor should be.

2.311 *His reputation is enhanced if he is quiet in manner and known to lead a regular life. He must be a gentleman, grave and kind to all.*

What a pity the expression "middle-class morality" cannot be emptied down the sluice where it belongs while the word gentleman is once more given its correct meaning severed from relationship with class, the highest compliment that can be paid to any man. The same goes for the word "lady". All doctors who follow the path of Hippocrates are ladies and gentlemen and it is probable they have been taught this from childhood whether their father was a bishop or what the sociologists politely call Social Class 5.

The last two requisites for studying medicine mentioned by Hippocrates are hard work and time. There is no escaping this. A medical student cannot become a good doctor without working for it any more than a fat person can become thin without dieting. This means isolation, poring over text books, drinking coffee to all hours and learning "the fifteen features" of thyrotoxicosis even if they are forgotten next day. However enthusiastic one is about vocational training, understanding the patient or peeling layers off onions, the whole lot are worthless without hard, grinding study. A doctor's job is medicine.

1.237 *The ability to study correctly what has been written by others is an important part of medicine. The man who learns and applies these will, I think, avoid serious mistakes.*

What is this ability to study correctly? We all have memories of turning over pages of text books without registering a single fact. We would not notice if we turned over two pages at once. This is a waste of time. The student has to lose himself in the text book just as he may lose himself in a novel, and because text books, unlike novels, tend to be boring this rarely happens. "Gray's Anatomy" does not often produce a state of bliss.

Correct study therefore demands special techniques and each student must devise what is best for himself. One obvious ploy is to read what he finds interesting, which usually means reading about a patient he has recently seen. This is being creative and the facts will probably stick because they form a pattern of which the patient may be a part.

If, as sometimes still happens to me in nightmares, I were to find myself once more sitting an exam, with the enemy facing me across the table, I would hope they would ask me about typhoid fever. This is because I have a clear typhoid Gestalt consisting of a particular patient, some extracts from a text book I read at the time with a few other oddments added later. I would pass with credit. But if, alas, the enemy asked me about cholera I would be finished. The cholera Gestalt consists of the phrase "rice-water" but I can never remember if this is what you give the patient to drink or if it is what comes out of his rectum.

Another device is for the student to ask himself questions as he goes along. This disturbs the flow but concentrates the attention. He covers sections of the text with his hand or a piece of paper and decides what he remembers about it. If the answer is "nothing" then he reads on and at least it will be like looking up answers to a crossword puzzle he cannot solve. If he does know something about the matter his knowledge is reinforced and added to. This is certainly more "correct study" than letting the words flow over him without any attempt to dam them. But whatever technique is used the cerebral cortex sets a time limit when, like Lashley's mice, he can no longer find his way through the maze. This is the time to do something else or go to bed.

1.329 *Experience is useful, the learning of other people's opinions far less so. For who would prefer clever argument to a calm and practised skill? So I advise you to listen to those who talk a lot but not to do what they say. They have an argumentative inefficiency, get angry and lack modesty, using definitions, assertions and oaths to prove their point. This may impress and bewilder the layman.*

This appears to be the reverse of the previous passage. The paradox is explained by the obvious fact that practice and learning go hand in hand. Both together lead to what we call experience. A book-learned doctor is not experienced, neither is a "barefoot doctor" who has treated a hundred cases of malaria but has never looked down a microscope. It is unrewarding to argue which is more important. They are complementary.

We have all met the sort of person Hippocrates mentions in the second half of this quotation. We learn to avoid them or do exactly the opposite of what they say. More dangerous are the subtle persuaders. The most obvious example is the worst sort of drug firm representative, happily a minority of those gallant people who sell their wares to doctors all over the world. He makes outrageous statements such as, "It is generally agreed that X is the best form of treatment for Y", when in fact the whole matter is controversial. He produces brightly coloured diagrams often in the form of blocks of which the bottom part has been lopped off to give an apparently sensational result:

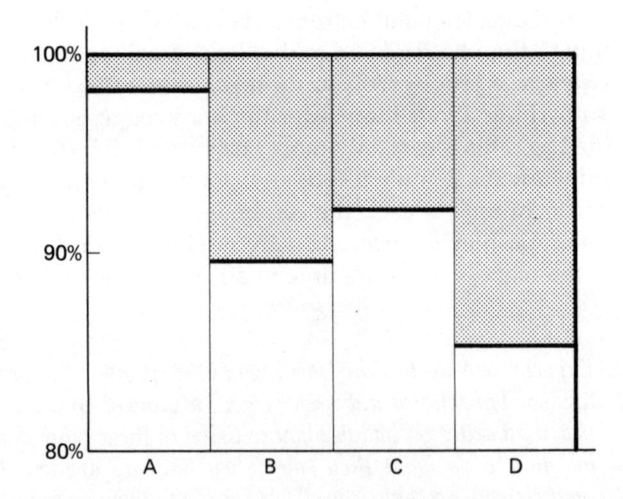

This diagram falsely suggests that A is five times more effective than D, which might as well be thrown in the dustbin even if it is ten times cheaper. There is a great art in transforming insignificant facts into significant pictures and most readers fall for it because the picture comes easier to the eye. It is a Gestalt which cheats the viewer.

Gifts, of course, help. The ball-point pen, the gadget for scraping frost off the car window, the dinner party or even the conference held near the golf course or palm-lined beach. Is this legitimate? It is certainly not a scientific way of deciding which product is best for the patient or cheapest for the tax-payer. Against this must be set the enormous help given by drug companies to education programmes. If doctors come to a lecture because the company provides nice sausage rolls they still benefit from the lecture although their motive in coming may be questioned.

2.265 *Inexperience is an accursed treasure; it is a stranger to confidence and joy and a nurse of cowardice and rashness. Cowardice indicates lack of will-power, rashness lack of art. There are in fact two things, science and opinion. The former begets knowledge, the latter ignorance.*

Inexperience is a disease all doctors suffer from. It is treatable but time is the chief factor in its cure and no-one can hurry time, although some educationalists think they can. Therefore it must be treated symptomatically and the best form of therapy is for the victim to realise how ignorant he is. Plato said, "One thing only I know and that is that I know nothing", and in a famous passage Newton wrote:

> "I do not know what I may appear to the world, but to myself I seem to have been only a boy playing on the seashore and diverting myself in now and then finding a smoother pebble or prettier shell than ordinary, whilst the great ocean of truth lay all undiscovered before me."

These admissions were made by two of the greatest thinkers of all time and this is one of the reasons for their greatness.

Hippocrates points out how a doctor can react inappropriately to the disease of inexperience. He can refrain from taking risks and learn nothing or he can rush in blindly and do enormous harm. This is why a good teacher is so important. He must have the skill gradually to withdraw as his pupil becomes more experienced until he finally becomes expendable himself. This requires a degree of modesty on the teacher's part. Without a teacher the pupil learns by his mistakes and this is not a good method, especially in the operating theatre. Doctors should learn *from* their mistakes, not *by* their mistakes, and there is a difference.

2.283 *The dominant factor is the personality . . . wisdom cannot be taught.*

This paraphrase sounds gloomy and is highly questionable. Wisdom is certainly more difficult to teach than knowledge but it grows with experience and with imitation of the wise. Otherwise why did Socrates or Plato or Hippocrates himself bother? However, medical students should be selected carefully with as much attention to their wisdom as their knowledge (exam results) because if there is little wisdom to start with growth will be slow. Nowadays this is generally accepted although tests of aptitude are not necessarily a better guide than general impressions or knowledge of the background. A doctor's son who is a good rugby player will probably turn out to be a good doctor, provided his cranium contains a reasonable number of cortical cells. This reactionary statement may produce jeers from the side-lines but it should at least be borne in mind alongside more scientific methods of appraisal which are sometimes a reflection of their creators rather than the student's worth.

A notable experiment took place at Cambridge in 1963 when students were given an ordinary examination paper and in addition an "alternative paper" devised to test imagination, or creativity as it is called today. The ones who did well in this paper did rather badly in the early part of the three year course but improved steadily until they got excellent degrees, comparable to those of scholars and exhibitioners.

These students were what we would nowadays call "divergers", in other words people who take a wide view of things, prefer to have a number of possible solutions to a problem, are not happy when tied down to facts and figures and do not mind an element of fantasy. They tend towards philosophy and the arts.

"Convergers" on the other hand like everything cut and dried. They prefer factual things and like a definitive answer. They are happy with measurements and numbers. And, mark this, they do well in exams in the earlier years of schooling. They are potential lords of the universe but their potentiality is not always fulfilled, because when it comes to higher academic grades and research the divergers overtake them.

The fallacy of this is that there is no such thing as a converger or a diverger. Each is a tendency, a phantom, and the purpose of this book is to show that a complete doctor must have within him both tendencies. To quote Liam Hudson, "He is involved in a choice among selves that already exist inside him". Clinical doctors especially should be human concertinas, converging and diverging at will. Because convergent factors are easy to study, books by the thousand are written about them. Books on divergent matters in medicine are few and far between. This is one of them, so it stands to reason that divergers will take to it more kindly than convergers.

2.281 *Be serious not devious, sharp witted, prepared to discuss and oppose those of like mind who are good tempered.*

What a superb definition of discussion as it should be! To be devious means to divert the argument into useless channels while at the same time looking intelligent. This may bring conversation to a halt with everyone baffled apart from the devious member who will appear the winner. The last sentence is vintage. "To oppose those of a like mind who are good tempered". When two or more people argue they should be on roughly the same level as each other, not too much above or too much below, and they must be confident the matter will not end in a shouting match, unless they happen to like shouting matches.

For many people discussion is the easiest way of learning because if it gets under way, it becomes enthralling. It is like a dinner party. The numbers must be right and the guests must be of comparable intellect but holding different views. Also, unlike a dinner party, there should be someone to keep order, otherwise as the enjoyment increases the learning value decreases. Next morning the guests will wake up and say to themselves, "That was a wonderful discussion. What on earth were we talking about?"

There is the other extreme. Some educators believe that comfortable discussion is of no value and "group leaders" should intentionally sow discord. It is only when there is conflict and discontent that learning gets under way. Some "refresher courses" are far from refreshing and I believe that where this doctrine is applied with lack of sensibility or lack of experience, the results for some people can be disastrous, for others boring or disillusioning. This applies especially to human relationship discussions which form an important part of training for general practice, but are largely neglected in hospitals where it is assumed that everyone gets on with everyone else and the doctors like the patients as much as the patients like the doctors. If a doctor has taken years to build up a form of defence around himself it is harmful to damage this unless it is done with tact, common sense and humour. It is equally harmful for a young doctor who has not yet organised his defences to be presented with fortifications which do not suit him.

Sadly, in some meetings or "modules" the ordinary courtesies seem to go by the board and there is little justification for this. There is no reason why discussions should not go to great depths and everyone be contented as well as enlightened. If the members of the discussion group are really upset that group should be counted a failure. This opinion which is, I believe, shared by most doctors who have been subjected to this kind of teaching, is a criticism of the extreme form of what is basically a good idea if carried out with "impartiality, propriety and modesty". Know thyself, but do not let thyself be torn to pieces.

A colleague of mine said to me the other day, "I think there are two important things in medicine – to know what you are doing and to do it kindly". Those who forget the second part are debasing the art of medicine and this applies to teaching as well as dealing with patients. Hippocrates, under his plane tree, would not have countenanced it.

2.279 *Any form of wisdom based on some scientific method is honourable, unless it is tainted with mere love of gain and unseemly behaviour. Such wisdom becomes popular through sheer impudence. The young become devotees of it, but when they are adult they become ashamed and when they are old they pass laws to banish it.*

This passage seems more applicable to politics than medicine. The young tend to seize on new and extravagant ideas and even support them with "unseemly behaviour". It is the teenagers who throw stones and terrorise the streets. In time they will grow out of this type of conduct even if they still support the idea. Later they grow out of the idea itself. This is one of the cycles of life. Can it be applied to medicine? Not perhaps to the medical student because he has to follow the precepts of his seniors and basically learn what they tell him to learn, otherwise he would not pass his exams or get a job.

It is relevant to groups of doctors working together, be it in a hospital unit or general practice. The fact of working together means they are learning from each other because they cannot do otherwise. The fascination of the situation is that each has a form of wisdom which is honourable but to some extent in conflict with the others. Because they are doctors, unseemly behaviour is frowned on, although love of gain is an important factor and not necessarily "mean".

Take as an example an imaginary partnership of general practitioners in England. There are, we will say, three doctors working in a practice in a health centre, which also lodges two other independent practices. The practices get on well together and there is a horizontal relationship between members of the same age group in the different practices. More important however is the vertical relationship of the three doctors who work together as a team. Each contributes his own brand of wisdom.

The older doctor has a close personal relationship with a relatively small number of patients whom he encourages to visit him frequently. They receive a good service and are dependent on the doctor's wisdom. He applies clinical medicine economically and rarely examines the patients. An occasional flick of the stethoscope is all they will get or want. The doctor has a lessening interest in the scientific aspects of the art although he tries to take an intelligent interest in them. His treatment is sometimes old fashioned yet in the partnership his wisdom is crucial.

The second doctor is at the height of his powers, having a blend of experience and knowledge of up-to-date medicine. He works quickly and efficiently. His wisdom lies in technique. Unless he has fallen by the wayside and become a cynic this technique will be backed by concern for his patients. If he has become a cynic or fails to learn from his partners, his powers will dwindle and his medicine become arid. At present he is the power-house of the practice.

The third doctor is younger and has the enthusiasm of new ideas. He is forever experimenting. Some experiments come off and some do not. His wisdom is a searching, creative mind. By definition he cannot attain what he seeks and this leads to frustration. At times he feels like putting a bomb under his partners, yet if he is wise himself he manages to control these feelings and learn from his partners' experience. His is the creative force and without him the practice will become stereotyped and go into decline.

This is a pattern which can be applied to many practices throughout the country and to any comparatively small group of doctors working together. It is, in modern parlance, a learning situation from which all partners should benefit provided the tensions are constructive rather than obstructive. Live and let live. Wisdom, technique and experiment are a good blend with rivalry adding a touch of piquancy.

The same pattern of behaviour can be applied to the individual doctor. His learning is a striving to balance these three factors within himself.

2.191 *It is a sign of a nasty nature or want of art to bring shame or abuse on the discoveries of others.*

When the tensions become too great jealousy is aroused. Doctors become critical of each other, either secretly or openly. Hippocrates' remark refers especially to doctors involved in research where there has to be rivalry. If controlled this is a stimulus, if uncontrolled – as in Hippocrates' reputed burning of the Cnidian library – obviously harmful. The Oxford–Cambridge, Harvard–Yale, Barts–Guys type of rivalry is excellent and finds some outlet in sport. If Oxford and Cambridge were to become departments of a single Combined University of Great Britain no-one would gain apart from those who find the Boat Race rather boring. Much would be lost and there is danger of research becoming a mammoth bureaucracy where individual ideas are stifled, and all the fun goes out of life.

Research workers require the modesty and generosity of an Isaac Newton. What worse fate can there be than to work for years on a project and find someone else publishing the results just before you do? Maybe the Cnidians discovered something which Hippocrates was on the point of publishing himself. However, rivals can be friendly. Wallace held an amicable correspondence with Darwin and, as far as I know, was not particularly upset when Darwin got the credit for the theory of evolution by natural selection. The Greeks who had thought it out 2,000 years before probably turned in their graves.

It has been pointed out that identical discoveries often take place in two places at the same time. Sometimes the names of the rivals are linked together in an eternal uneasy wedlock, like "Plummer and Vinson" which, after research by purists, was reversed into "Vinson and Plummer". Later purists found earlier descriptions of the syndrome and called it the Patterson–Kelly or Kelly–Patterson syndrome, later adding the third name of Brown, making it into the Patterson–Kelly–Brown syndrome. This makes nonsense of medical indexing as well as confusing the student. Nonetheless a discoverer should have his reward and I always prefer to use the term Crohn's disease to regional ileitis. I also find an expression like "Charcot's intermittent hepatic fever'' rolls off the tongue so smoothly that it has a poetic value and I use it in preference to recurrent cholangitis. Tic Douloureux too is an expression that should not be lost. Although Trigeminal Neuralgia is more scientifically accurate it does not express the feelings of the patient, of which the doctor should be constantly reminded.

Determination to defeat rivals can lead to cheating and there have been unfortunate cases of this sort. Recently the statistical results of a well-known survey were shown to work out exactly right, which is itself a statistical impossibility. The only explanation was that the sums were done backwards starting with the results.

This sort of thing usually occurs with scientists who have made their reputation and feel they cannot afford to be wrong, rather like Mediums who lose their psychic powers and start blowing cheese-cloth out of the various orifices of their body. The most famous example was Charles Dawson who hoaxed anthropologists with the Piltdown Man by staining a mixed assortment of bones. The same thing can occur in medicine. Although there was probably no conscious cheating involved we blush to think of the number of total dental extractions performed to eliminate toxic substances from the blood because of someone's unintelligent guess work. Circumcision and tonsillectomy come into a similar category, although there was again no intentional cheating but possibly ''a mean love of gain''. How many more medical skeletons will rise from their graves?

Personal rivalry is rife in hospital. One well-known physician used to refer to his even more famous colleague as ''my assistant in the electrocardiographic department''. I have seen rival surgical teams passing each other in the corridor with heads averted, starting with the chief surgeon in the front and finishing with the junior student in the rear. Such behaviour brings ridicule on the medical profession. As has been said in an earlier chapter, the worst fault of all is for a doctor to be critical of another doctor in front of a patient.

1.323 *To be jealous is a sign of weakness and more suitable to the market place than medicine.*

It is also a handicap to education because the student or young doctor involved in this sort of rivalry will have a biased view of the subject. He will be led to believe that one particular form of treatment is right, the rest wrong; one operation is *the* operation.

2.285 *To have ideas without putting them into action is a sign of inadequate education and inadequate understanding of the art.*

This refers to book learning unrelated to the patient. It was mentioned in an earlier chapter that disease does not exist on its own. No-one, apart from a pathologist, can study coronary thrombosis without it being attached to a living patient, and once it is so attached it becomes part of a complex of attitudes and emotions. This is well illustrated in the following case history which showed an inadequate understanding of the art.

Case 48 A man of 68 was brought to a doctor's surgery in his daughter's car, where he was seen by a relatively inexperienced doctor. He had suffered from a bout of chest pain 48 hours previously, which had lasted three hours. He had felt sick and vomited once with some relief. The pain had not recurred. The delay in the visit was due to the daughter telling the receptionist on the 'phone that her father was getting indigestion, without mentioning this particular attack of chest pain. He had therefore been given an appointment for two days later. The doctor examined the patient and, although he could find no abnormality, considered that he might have had a coronary thrombosis. This was a justifiable assumption but what happened later was questionable. The doctor, "doing it by the book", told the patient he had had a heart attack. He was required to remain lying on the couch until an ambulance arrived. Although the patient had walked up a flight of stairs to the consulting room, the ambulance men were instructed to carry him downstairs on a stretcher. The patient was taken to a hospital where an electrocardiogram was done. This was normal. A more careful history showed that the chest pain had come on soon after the patient had eaten a plate of pork and chips and had been intermittent in intensity. The doctor could hardly be faulted on technical grounds, because prolonged chest pain is a coronary thrombosis until proved otherwise and the patient appeared to be at risk from cardiac arrhythmia.

However, he misjudged the situation, that is to say, the disease in relation to the patient. This was a man of 68 with a history of chest pain 48 hours previously. The chance of arrhythmia was remote and a man of that age would probably do better at home than in hospital. If an ECG was considered necessary the daughter could well have driven him to the hospital without fuss or taken him home to bed where a domicillary ECG could have been arranged.

As it was, the surgery session was completely disrupted and the patient, having been told he had a heart attack and having been treated in such a dramatic way, quite naturally refused to believe his heart was normal. His daughter, who was emotionally unstable, reinforced this view, and the patient became a cardiac cripple. This was a disaster due to inappropriate action by the doctor. He failed to balance the pros and cons, although, if the unlikely had happened, a coroner would have supported his action.

2.227 *It is difficult to find out about the failings of medicine, easier to find out the successes. The layman cannot determine the failures but the skilled physician can, because they are matters of understanding rather than physical results.*

The case just described was a dismal failure. Yet the doctor concerned probably did not realise it to be so, especially as he was not responsible for the later care of the patient. The "physical results" were satisfactory because a patient who might have died of coronary thrombosis did not do so. The failure then was a "matter of understanding". This is where a good teacher comes in. It is the most difficult task of the teacher to point out the mistakes of his pupil particularly if that pupil is also a colleague. With medical students the problem is less because they are expected to make mistakes and tolerate harsh criticism. The best teacher I ever had was a master of sarcasm, and I found it hard to sleep the night before his notorious Friday teaching round, when the students were arraigned before an audience of postgraduate enthusiasts. He was, incidentally a kind-hearted man.

Once the student is qualified he becomes a colleague, that is to say an equal. But, to use yet another variation on a well known dictum, all doctors are equal but some doctors are more equal than others. It is the duty of the teacher not only to point out errors but to seek them avidly. Mistakes that remain hidden tend to fester, that is to say become habits. How can a teacher do this without becoming a tyrant, or worse still, a nagger?

The first essential is a good relationship, that is to say one of mutual respect. The second is an agreement on both strategy and tactics at the start of the campaign. The type of campaign I am experienced in is the teaching of general practice, where the trainee is in an anomalous position of being responsible for the care of his patients as a qualified doctor and at the same time responsible to his trainer for doing this in a reasonably efficient manner. What an opportunity for friction and how rarely it occurs!

The strategy is that the trainer has a right to check the work of the trainee either with the previous knowledge of both or as a spot check, *provided* the trainee can do the same to the trainer in return. The tactics are as follows, and this an entirely personal way of working.

1. The trainer and trainee do a surgery together each week, the trainer being in the hot seat one week, the trainee the next. Whoever is in charge will decide which consultation will be a two-way affair between himself and the patient, with the other doctor a spectator (or spectre) in the background, and which will be a three-way discussion. This sounds a very traumatic procedure for all concerned but it is not so in practice. Each consultation falls into a natural pattern and there is rarely embarrassment. The patients usually preferred this to an ordinary consultation because they found the atmosphere more friendly and they were getting better attention. Two for the price of one. Of course as soon as each patient leaves the room the spectre in the background is at liberty to criticise both the technique and clinical skill of his colleague. This is the only way I know of studying how a doctor does his work, without using complex apparatus such as one way mirrors or videotape. An audiotape is not of much

value since it fails to record vital non-verbal messages transmitted between patient and doctor. Besides all these present ethical problems in relation to confidentiality.

2. The trainer and trainee pick out case notes at random, look at each other's notes and in thirty seconds try to extract as much information as possible. They then criticise the content and legibility.
3. The trainer and trainee quiz each other either on subjects prepared in advance or on random topics. We use a technique called Party Games. A pack of cards is prepared on each of which is written a problem. The doctor selects a card and has to give an immediate answer. This simulates a surgery situation and makes it more exciting for both doctors, because neither knows which card will turn up. The problems can be about anything clinical or nonclinical, simple or complicated. Here are some examples.

   A girl of fifteen sits down in front of you and says in a matter of fact way, "I want an abortion". What would you do?

   Your receptionist 'phones you. She is obviously angry and upset. She says there is a patient in the waiting room who insists on seeing you at once. He has had a cough for a week. When she offered him an appointment for tomorrow he became abusive. What would you do?

   A mother brings a baby of four months to the surgery. Your partner had seen her the day before and prescribed a mixture for a cold. The mother says the baby is worse and while she is talking to you the baby starts having a fit. What would you do?

These are all situations which put the doctor on the spot. They require an immediate decision of some kind and are just the sort of incidents which do occur.

The three methods of assessment which have been described are used for checking the trainee's style of medicine as well as his clinical knowledge which can be tested by the standard type of questions, written or oral. The important thing to find out is how the trainee applies his knowledge.

Hospital medicine and general practice differ in many respects. In some ways it is easier to check the work of a junior doctor in a hospital training post because the illness is not such an individual matter between him and the patient, and much of what he does is seen or discussed by his seniors. However I think the same principle holds. No senior doctor should teach or criticise a junior doctor unless he allowed himself to be open to criticism of a similar kind. The autocratic teacher has probably outlived his day, although I remember him with respect and nostalgia.

1.327 *If you wish to give a lecture to impress a crowded audience your ambition is not praiseworthy. At least avoid citations from the poets because to quote them argues feeble composition. For I forbid in medical practice a craft not pertinent to the Art but laboriously far-fetched, but which has in itself an attractive grace. For you will achieve the empty toil of a drone and a drone's spoils.*

Mea culpa! Of course I do not agree with Hippocrates on this point because my theme is that sensibility, in which I include poetry and art, is an important ingredient of medicine. I hope he is referring to those highly rhetorical lecturers who impress their audience but teach them nothing. "More matter with less art", as Hamlet's mother said impatiently to Polonius. In my experience the opposite type of lecturer is more common, one who presents facts but in such an unpalatable form that the listener can neither swallow nor digest them. The number of facts which can be absorbed in a given time are anyway small and if they have no emotional attachment they become infinitesimal. Humour, too, is important. I think that the essential thing is that art and matter should be combined in the right proportion and be relevant to each other. It amazes me that lecturers in medicine have practically no training in the art of lecturing. It is assumed that if they have a medical degree they must be able to teach, and if they understand the complexities of their subject they can, as a matter of course, lucidly explain these complexities to other people. I hope the time will come when any doctor who takes a post in which teaching or lecturing are important will be required to undertake training or even pass an exam in the art of teaching.

2.281 *Setting out in effective language what has been shown, graceful in speech, gracious in disposition, with a reputation for supporting the truth.*

This is more like the ideal teacher. The expression "effective language" is important. This implies using words which mean what they say and are understood by the listener. It excludes on the one hand woolliness and on the other hand jargon, the two cardinal sins of both speaking and writing.

2.193 *For names are conventions but real essences are not conventions but the offspring of nature.*

Words are very important. They are not the essence of meaning but they convey the essence either well or badly. T. S. Eliot put the matter concisely when he described a well-written or well-spoken sentence,

> ". . . where every word is at home,
> Taking its place to support the others,
> The word neither diffident nor ostentatious,
> An easy commerce of the old and the new,
> The common word exact without vulgarity,
> The formal word precise but not pedantic,
> The complete consort dancing together. . . ."

Today there is a sad tendency to use jargon, and by jargon I imply words that mean less, not more than the words they replace but at the same time lack precision. They stultify thought because they are repetitive and give an illusion of cleverness. Take the following statement by a Trades' Union Shop Steward: "At this moment in time all I can say is that at shop floor level we seek wage differentials and job satisfaction. There is still room for manoeuvre and at the grass roots we hope to avoid escalation and confrontation with management and get round the table to formulate a productivity scheme within the guidelines." This is, in fact, a sensible or "meaningful" statement but it is so incredibly boring that the listener is either lulled to sleep or unfairly antagonised. We have heard it all before.

In medicine, jargon is not only boring but incomprehensible to all except the initiated few and I am not referring to essential technical terms for specialist readers. Those who use jargon are mostly the organisers or administrators and they tend to become cut off from their colleagues, the grass-roots if you like, simply because these colleagues do not know what they are talking about. And why should they? If information is to be passed to "ordinary doctors", that is 90% of the total, it should be in current medical language. Throw in a few words like feed-back, input, paradigm, modality; add some unknown initials such as W.P.P. (which stands for Whole Person Pathology) or a distorted word or two from the classics such as "aegis"; include the suffix -situation after as many expressions as possible, such as the "family-situation", and the lecturer might as well go home or the article not be written. Those who wish to explore this matter further should read Madden's essay in the journal World Medicine of September 7th, 1977 which has a sub-title "If it's worth saying at all, it's worth saying offensively". I have borrowed some of these expressions from this essay and there are many more.

There is, of course, a counter-argument that the vocabulary is valuable and should be learnt by all up-to-date doctors. I do not believe this to be so, largely because it is condemned by its own ugliness, but also because it detracts from personal relationships in the guise of explaining them. It may have value as a research tool but not in the "feed-back communication situation".

1.299 *I will respect my teacher as I would my parents and will ensure he is adequately rewarded and will pass on his teaching to others in my profession.*

This comes opportunely after the previous diatribe. A teacher should be respected but, for this, he must be understood and it is the doctor's responsibility to pass on his teaching to others if it is of value. This excerpt is a paraphrase of part of the Hippocratic Oath. In the original version the pupil was required to support his teacher financially.

1.299 *. . . to make him partner in my livelihood: where he is in need of money to share mine with him.*

This would not be a very popular idea today. In Hippocrates' time the teacher and his pupils were part of an "extended family", studying, living and eating together. The teacher thus became a foster father and family obligations applied.

The paraphrased version is highly relevant today. Teachers in most countries are poorly paid in relation to their skills. University lecturers or professors are in general paid less than practical clinicians, a strange situation if it is assumed that a teacher should be superior to his pupil. The other point Hippocrates makes is that doctors should be responsible for payment of the profession as a whole, not only for themselves. If a class of doctors is underpaid the profession should see that justice is done. It is also their concern if patients are overcharged or exploited. However, doctors individually and as a profession should behave with dignity and restraint because Hippocratic ideals apply to this as much as to behaviour with patients. If they use doubtful or harmful methods they will lose all rights to a privileged status.

10

The Art and the Mind

2.175 *Men ought to know that from the brain, and the brain only, arise our pleasures, joys, laughter and jokes, as well as our sorrows, pains, grief and tears. Through our brains we see, hear and distinguish the ugly from the beautiful, the bad from the good, the pleasant from the unpleasant. Sometimes we decide from our own experience, sometimes from the natural value of the matter.*

This is for me one of the finest passages in the Collection. It is near to poetry. Inside every Hippocrates there is a Euripides struggling to get out.

These words were written some two thousand years before their time. It is only comparatively recently that the brain has been accepted as the sole organ of awareness and perception. We still talk of people being warm-hearted, lily-livered, and having no stomach for a fight. If we go to church the priest may gloss over the word "bowels" while reading the epistle for the day. Oliver Cromwell wrote "I beseech you, in the bowels of Christ . . ." and those were powerful words.

It is easy to understand how this error appeared in Hippocrates' time. Although the brain is our source of pleasure, pain and so on, it is the mistress of the whole body and uses other organs to express its feelings. "Having no stomach for the fight" is a good description of the sinking feeling experienced before battle or sitting an exam; the lover's heart reacts strongly to the sight of the loved one and there was no reason to think of the brain as a go-between.

2.181 *Some people say the heart is the organ with which we think and it feels pain and anxiety. But it is not so.*

Now we know better and are even able to stop ourselves shaking and quaking by swallowing B-blocker tablets before making an after-dinner speech or taking a driving test. These are not tranquillisers. They suppress the physical symptoms of anxiety which can be embarrassing.

The brain is the person, the rest of the body appendages. A patient is thought of as being dead when the electroencephalogram shows no activity, even when the appendages are functioning normally. It is theoretically possible to perfuse a human head with no body attached and have a living person. I have seen this portrayed in a late night horror film on television and it was something I did not quickly forget.

2.179 *I consider the brain the most powerful organ of the human body for when it is healthy it acts as an interpreter of the phenomena of the outside world. Eyes, ears, tongue, hands and feet obey the brain in its discernment of these things. The brain is the messenger of consciousness.*

The expression "when it is healthy" bring us at once into difficulties. When is the brain, or mind, healthy? At what point do we call a patient mentally ill? How much mental illness should a doctor allow his patient? A lot of nonsense has been written about this but as a practising family doctor I accept two criteria for mental illness.

If the patient is unhappy and this unhappiness is out of proportion to the cause or is prolonged far beyond what is reasonable, then I call the patient mentally ill. If a patient behaves in a way which is in conflict with his environment and is not acceptable to other people, then again I would call him mentally ill.

No precise definition is possible. If the environment itself is ill then the patient might be called normal. A hippie is normal amongst hippies and a psychopath normal on the staff of a concentration camp. Also the decision depends on the person making it, his upbringing, his tolerance and his mood of the moment. After a ghastly surgery a doctor may say to his receptionist, "What a load of neurotics we had this evening", thereby making a not very good judgement of their mental state. If he was in a good mood he would consider them normal people with problems, and might have enjoyed working through some of the problems with them.

Broadly speaking the first criterion includes patients with chronic or severe anxiety or depression, and those with more serious illnesses such as schizophrenia or dementia but with enough insight to realise they are miserable. The second criterion includes patients who lack insight, such as the severely schizophrenic or demented and some psychopaths who think they are right and the rest of the world is wrong. The two criteria are not necessarily exclusive and a patient may flit between one and the other, as John Clare did.

Case 49 A man of 70, an author of some repute, found his mental powers were waning. He was commissioned to write a book but found he could spend a morning in his study without putting a word on paper. This was the onset of senile dementia and his consciousness of this made him depressed and irritable. He was clearly mentally ill by the first criterion.

A small stroke accelerated his dementia. He lost insight and ceased to worry about his writing and about his own illness. He became placid and easy to manage. As the dementia progressed he was admitted to a mental hospital where he was happy because he believed he was back in his old university college. Provided he was allowed to sit at the "high table" for meals he had no quarrel with the other "dons" and was well treated by the college porters (nurses). He was now mentally ill by the second criterion because his behaviour would have been unacceptable and distressing outside a mental hospital. He passed his time happily with this and other delusions, apart from very occasional intrusions into reality, until he died peacefully of pneumonia.

The writings of Laing and his colleagues have become popular in recent years and have brought about a new attitude to mental illness. Laing considers that schizophrenia does not exist as an entity but is a fabrication of the psychiatrist's mind in relation to certain situations, especially family conflicts. In an earlier chapter it was pointed out that no disease exists on its own, be it pneumonia or schizophrenia, but it simply will not do to deny that patients present with symptoms which can usefully be called schizophrenic. Over and over again I have seen this pattern and, although the Gestalt is compounded partly from what I have read in books, I would refute that it is a fabrication. The definition is important because the treatment of schizophrenia is different from that of a psychoneurosis and on the whole successful. The diagnosis is necessary as a practical matter.

I admire Laing's sympathy for schizophrenic patients and his realisation that their madness contains truth if the doctor is prepared to listen. There is method in their madness as indeed in all madness. No spoken word or action arises from nothing even if the sequence is illogical to everyone save the patient.

Some may be happy with their mild schizophrenic state and can be safely allowed to get on with it, but if they cross the barriers of the two criteria I have mentioned, namely unhappiness or incompatability with society, they deserve treatment. In my opinion treatment implies physical treatment because no-one can talk himself out of a schizophrenic state. As Laing himself says, these patients are more afraid of being understood than misunderstood.

The following case shows how one is groping in the dark with mental illness. It perhaps contradicts what I have just written.

Case 50 Marjorie S. was an unfortunate person. The youngest and plainest of a family of four girls, she was so shy as a child that she could not talk to anyone without holding her hands in front of her face. Her three sisters married young and left home, so Marjorie stayed to look after her ageing parents. As an adult she was as unprepossessing as she had been as a child and the pattern of her life seemed assured. The doctor rarely saw her but whenever he did he was vaguely worried. However there seemed to be nothing he could do about the situation.

One day he was surprised to catch a glimpse from his car window of her walking arm-in-arm with a young man and was even more surprised a few weeks later to read the announcement of her engagement in a local paper. She brought her fiancé to the surgery. He seemed an uncouth person but the doctor congratulated them, feeling that "beggars can't be choosers".

A few months after the wedding Marjorie came to the surgery and shyly admitted she might be pregnant. This was confirmed by a pregnancy test and she was delighted. Her personality seemed to change, presumably because she had something to live for after so many years of discouragement. She attended the surgery frequently just to talk about the coming baby and her manner was now vivacious.

She had an easy confinement but unfortunately the baby was born with a port-wine stain on the side of the face, extending half-way down the thorax. When Marjorie was shown the baby she pushed him away and burst into tears. After this it was a long uphill struggle. The husband was not much help because, for some reason, he thought the defect in the baby was Marjorie's fault. Gradually however they both came to accept the situation and Marjorie went to the other extreme and became over-possessive towards the child. No-one, not even her husband, was allowed to feed the baby and she resented any interference from the doctor or health visitor.

When the child was eight months old he had a major fit and developed hemiplegia. He was admitted to hospital where a diagnosis of Sturge Weber syndrome was made, namely an intracerebral haemangioma associated with the port-wine stain of the skin. This presumably had bled and unfortunately the hemiplegia was permanent.

Marjorie's reaction to all this was puzzling. She showed little emotion when it was explained to her that her son would grow up paralysed on one side. She took

> the child home and carried out her duties as a mother efficiently but rather mechanically. A few months later it was reported to the doctor that Marjorie was behaving in a peculiar way. She was stopping people in the street and asking them to admire her child, thereby causing much embarrassment. She had also put his name down for a famous public school which anyway she could not afford.
>
> The doctor found a pretext for visiting the house and it was clear that Marjorie's behaviour was paranoid. She had decided her son was going to be a football player and had already written to the manager of a well-known club. She had also written to the B.B.C. because she had decided he was going to be a television announcer. She lived in a world of fantasy but appeared to carry on her household duties reasonably well. Her husband's attitude was casual. He did not bother to listen to her and as long as he got his meals regularly he did not seem to mind.
>
> A psychiatrist was asked to see her and after much discussion it was decided best to give her a monthly injection of Fluphenazine. Hospital admission was considered unnecessary but it was thought that she would not take tablets regularly and her husband could not be relied on to see she did and this was the reason for giving injections.
>
> The treatment worked. Her fantasy world evaporated. She became quieter and ceased to talk about her extravagant plans for the child. Four months later she committed suicide.

This affair raises questions which are difficult to answer. It could be that her fantasies were necessary for her survival and she was deprived of these by the treatment. The world was so harsh that she needed to be a paranoid schizophrenic to live in it. The doctor had overstepped the mark in treating her. On the other hand, by the previous criterion, her behaviour was becoming unacceptable to other people and would probably have become worse. Either way the doctor could have been wrong.

This case has been set out at length because I consider it important. It gives some support for Laing's theories. However, it is a single example of failure in treatment and must be put beside many successes where the patient has returned to his ordinary life.

Laing's ideas travel light-years beyond this. They become more and more complex and could do with a good douche of common sense from time to time. The same goes for many theoretically minded psychiatrists, who are positively frightened by the simple truth and feverishly set about complicating it. A spider's web is beautiful because of its simplicity. If the spider were to keep on adding extra strands it would be a mess and would incidentally fail to catch flies. Spiders are sensible creatures. So were the Greeks. They, too, believed in symmetry and simplicity.

Psychiatric theory can go deeper and deeper until even the poor foetus is not immune from emotional stresses. Medawar expressed this neatly when he talked of psychiatrists who "like sloshing about in amniotic fluid". Superficial interpretations should not be ignored and I like the following passage written by Julian Mitchell:

> "Freud is all nonsense; the secret of neurosis is to be found in the family battle of wills to see who can refuse longest to help with the dishes. The sink is the great symbol of the bloodiness of family life. All life is bad but family life is worse."

Laing's great contribution has been his sympathy with the feelings of the mentally ill and by this I mean true "poetic" understanding as opposed to distant kindness. He would have got on well with John Clare. I wonder if he realises that Euripides, Hippocrates' alter ego, expressed the same feelings 2,400 years ago? In an amazing play "Heracles", or "Hercules Furens" to give it its Latin title, he introduces Madness as a person. The messenger of the gods Iris obeys her mistress Hera (Juno) and brings Madness to Hercules, but Madness, being tolerant by nature, does not wish to inflict herself on him.

"My nature's noble as my parents were,
Heaven my father, night my mother."

"I only thought how I might turn your
path towards good instead of evil."

To which Iris replies irritably,

"The Queen of Heaven did not send you here to think."

So Madness, against her better judgment, takes control of Hercules.

"I'll plague you worse yet. You shall dance
in terror to my piping."

Hercules in his frenzy kills his own children and the only light in the ghastly tragedy is the compassion he receives from his friend Theseus. No psychiatry here, just friendship.

The expression "Heaven my father, night my mother" is worth considering. What an extraordinary thing to say about madness! It is another way of putting what John Clare and others have said. If turned towards good, Madness is creativeness, fantasy, sensibility; if towards bad, it is nightmare and misery. It is a distortion of personality not something new in itself.

2.175 *It is the brain also which makes us mad or delirious, inspires us with dread or fear by night and day, causes sleeplessness, unfortunate mistakes, unnecessary anxiety, absent-mindedness and unusual behaviour.*

What a superb comprehensive description of mental illness! Here we have the simplicity of the spider's web. Most of the incidents of madness described by Hippocrates were forms of delirium caused by acute and often fatal infections. He did not seem to distinguish these from madness of other kinds and the description below would do for either.

1.283 *The wife of Delearches was seized after grief with an acute fever and shivering. From the start she wrapped herself up and throughout, without speaking a word, would fumble, pluck, scratch, pick hairs, weep and then laugh, but she did not sleep.*

But in the following passages he seems to realise the importance of depression as an illness.

4.191 *Delirium with laughter is less dangerous than delirium with seriousness.*

4.185 *Prolonged fear or depression means melancholia.*

In his day psychiatry was not, it seems, a recognised branch of medicine. Mental illness was more the province of the priest. In some passages of the Collection Hippocrates appears to confuse it with epilepsy but in the following extract he makes a distinction. It is not clear however if he considered madness to be a disease as such or ill-health caused by human or divine pressures. We still do not know the answer to that one.

2.139 *I am going to discuss epilepsy, the disease called "sacred". It is no more sacred than any other disease but has a natural cause. Its supposed sacredness is due to man's ignorance and his wonder at its unusual character. If it is considered sacred just because it is extraordinary then any extraordinary disease should be called sacred, such as malaria and some forms of madness.*

Divine or natural, the two meant the same to Hippocrates, so it is what we would call nowadays a "non-question". Hippocrates is sarcastic about the idea that different symptoms can be attributed to "possession" by different gods.

2.147 *If the patient imitate a goat, if he roar or suffer convulsions on the right side they say Hera, the Mother of the Gods, is to blame.*

When at night occur fears and terrors, delirium, jumpings from the bed and rushings out of doors, they say that Hecate is attacking.

And on a more ridiculous plane –

2.147 *If the faeces are more frequent and thinner, like that of birds, it is Apollo Nomius.*

This is fame for Apollo Nomius, who might have got his name in the textbooks like Dr Crohn of Crohn's disease. Hippocrates had little to say about treatment, except he mentions the drug Hellebore as being useful in mental disease. Opiates and alcohol were no doubt widely used for anxiety and mania.

1.331 *Some people are upset and grieve over the troubles of others. Loud talking distresses them. They should be persuaded from overactivity. A wooded district is helpful.*

Anxiety states and a wish to "get away from it all" are nothing new. Woods and forests are still popular places for peace and quiet. So is the seaside. The Greeks found the "wine-dark sea" unpredictable and frightening. It conjured up shipwreck and strange monsters who would be quite capable of creeping up the beach and snatching sunbathers, had the Greeks ever considered seaside holidays as a profitable pastime.

4.257 *Change and variation give most pleasure. If a musician composed a tune on one note it would give no pleasure at all.*

Boredom was one of the greatest enemies of happiness to the Greeks as it is to us. It is sometimes forgotten that Athens and Cos were slave societies where the rich had little to do apart from attending the gymnasium or gossiping, unless there was a war on the go when their energies were consumed in military activities. Life for the women must have been very drab. They were a subjugated class and were not even allowed to sit at the dinner table when guests were invited. They probably enjoyed running the household and were often skilled in feminine occupations such as weaving. It must have been a real day out to go to the theatre, which was intensely exciting. It is said that at a performance of one play of Aeschylus the audience were so terrified that several women had miscarriages on the spot.

It is the dramatists who tell us more about mental illness because in each play there is at least one character who is, to put it mildly, unstable. Little is said about treatment apart from purification or atonement for past wrongs, either the patient's own or his ancestors'. Orestes, having murdered his mother Clytemnestra, was pursued relentlessly by the Furies (his own guilt) from land to land until he at last found peace and reason in the tolerant atmosphere of Athens. It was these Furies in fact who caused the outbreak of miscarriages, already mentioned, in the theatre at Athens.

In a slightly less traumatic situation such as occurred in Euripides' "Medea", where the heroine was insanely, but justifiably, jealous of another woman for whom her husband had deserted her, the Chorus gave advice of a rather half-hearted nature.

> "Will she listen when we are speaking
> To the word we say?
> I wish she might relax her rage
> And temper of her heart."

The Chorus, like all good psychiatrists, gave Medea plenty of scope to talk about her problems but this merely added fuel to the flames. Medea became so embittered that she murdered not only her rival but her own children whom she loved. In this she showed a "divided self". Such incidents are occasionally reported in the newspapers of today. It must have been quite obvious to the Chorus that the correct treatment for Medea was restraint in an institution for the protection of the public. Unfortunately, by convention, the Chorus was not permitted to influence the action of the play so they could do little but bewail what was going on.

This is all very well. Aeschylus, Sophocles and Euripides give us remarkable insight into the human mind but no practical instruction to the doctor faced with a mentally ill patient. Let us therefore be practical and discuss what can be done to help the mentally ill patient of today.

For myself, as a family doctor, there seem to be three forms of available treatment which, for the sake of simplicity, I will call the short interview, the long interview and physical treatment, which means drugs and such activities as electroconvulsive therapy. The complete doctor, be he a psychiatrist or not, should have expertise in all three methods, because each is relevant to particular patients. To choose the wrong treatment can be just as damaging as failing to diagnose an acute abdomen. Tragically many doctors become obsessed with one approach to treatment and use this to the exclusion of others. This is often because they belong to a particular school. When someone mentions the word "school" I feel like Goering who said, "When I hear of anyone talk of Culture I reach for my gun". It implies that the doctor is limiting himself to one aspect of human nature. He denies himself the chance to take a broad view of the patient, the sort of view which would be taken by a good novelist or indeed by an ordinary human being. He is therefore shutting himself off from part of reality either because he has been indoctrinated by his seniors or because he is incapable of facing up to reality himself. Fortunately schools of psychology are going out of fashion, even if dogma is not. The best description I know of the dangers of dogmatic thinking is contained in Axel Munthe's classic "The Story of San Michele". He describes in horrifying detail Charcot's demonstrations of hypnotic behaviour and *grande hystérie* at the Salpêtrière, the whole wretched affair being a Gestalt of Charcot's own creation. He made his patients fit the Gestalt to their own disadvantage but to his intellectual gain and to the amusement of the public. The patients became performing animals.

1.15 *The exponent of an insoluble mystery must use a postulate, for*

> *example things in the sky or below the earth. If a man were to learn or declare the state of these it would not be clear if his statement were true either to himself or his audience. For there is no test whose application would give proof.*

This admirably describes the quandary of psychiatry today. The human mind is an insoluble mystery so we have to seek explanations which are, at least in part, symbolic. We like to think they are scientific but we are wrong if we do because, as Karl Popper has pointed out, there is no means of *disproving* psychiatric theory. No-one can refute Freud's theories, nor for that matter Adler's or Jung's or anyone else's. What I wrote about the family role-playing of the doctor is also irrefutable but this does not mean it is necessarily true. Psychiatric theory is therefore more akin to philosophy and religion than to science. The attempts to fit it into a scientific mould are doomed from the start, providing only information on side issues.

But to return to the main issue, namely treatment of mental illness – the short interview is the technique most commonly used because of its brevity. It is employed by all doctors and one must presume Hippocrates was a master of it. The surgeon who bothers to find out that his patient is worried and says "The operation is my worry not yours" is using this form of treatment. A patient about to have an operation is like a passenger in an aeroplane. If anything goes wrong he can do nothing about it so he might as well sit back and leave it to the pilot.

The family doctor is the pastmaster at this art, partly because he probably knows the patient already so does not have to start laboriously at the beginning; partly because time compels him to work out a short interview technique for himself. It is important that time should be the doctor's ally, not his enemy. If ten minutes is the allotted time he should do his best in ten minutes and not bewail the fact that he cannot have half an hour. After all it would be just as bad if it was the other way round and he had to give a ten-minute patient half an hour. Think of all the onion layers he would be compelled to peel off in this time!

The art of the short interview is to get to the point quickly, using at times what Balint's colleagues call the "flash technique", that is to say intuition based on experience. The other important point is for the doctor to make the patient realise he is on his side. This can be done by using simple expressions such as "I don't know how you stick it" or "I expect that infuriates you". It is sometimes a good plan to anticipate what the patient is going to say by putting the words into his mouth. For example if a mother is obviously irritated by her child the consultation might go something like this:

Doctor: And I expect you feel like chucking him out of the window sometimes?
Patient: That's just it.
Doctor: Then one feels guilty afterwards.
Patient: I feel so ashamed about it.
Doctor: You needn't. It happens to all of us. I often used to feel like strangling my children. But I loved them all the same. What particular things irritate you?

The doctor is sharing his patient's feelings and it must be remembered that some aunt or other has previously told her these feelings are "unnatural". The consultation will last a few more minutes and the doctor may or may not give her some practical advice on how to escape from the constant presence of her child and he may or may not prescribe a mild tranquilliser. I usually ask to see the patient a fortnight later and am amazed how helpful this kind of treatment is. The patient has really wanted *someone* to understand her. It is better to avoid large doses of antidepressants or tranquillisers initially because they will very likely make the patients feel ill, just after the doctor has promised to make them feel better. This is like a slap on the face after a handshake.

The short interview can be repeated indefinitely but the doctor should beware of this. If the patient attends three times or more he is on the way to becoming a chronic attender, a difficult state of affairs when a doctor may have to see the patient at regular intervals year after year long after they have run out of conversation. If the short interviews fail it is better to arrange a long interview and get down to some real onion-peeling. The doctor can then decide his course of action. The decision may be not to see the patient any more, if possible, because neither of the participants will benefit from the relationship.

Usually however the doctor should leave himself available on demand, especially if there is an inescapable situation such as awkward elderly parents or a drunken husband. It is often enough for the patient just to know the doctor is there; he hardly ever needs to visit and this is very economical in time. If the doctor blatantly rejects the patient he is building up trouble for himself or his partners. The patient will probably realise that he will get nowhere with psychological illness and resort to spurious physical symptoms until everyone is driven to distraction.

Of course many anxious patients present with physical illness. The experienced doctor will probably get an almost instantaneous "flash" but should not insult the patient by failing to carry out a reasonable examination. He can then put his short interview technique into operation.

I have often heard the short interview technique denigrated but it follows the precept of Hippocrates.

3.383 *What you should put first in all the practice of our art is to make the patient well; and if he can be made well in many ways choose the least troublesome.*

There is often a fear in the doctor's mind that a patient with recurrent vague symptoms may have some hidden organic disease, even if his initial "flash" has been supported by a long tale of woes. Strangely enough it is considered a heinous offence for a doctor to mistake a physical illness for an emotional one. The other way round is bad luck or the patient's fault.

If a physical cause seems likely the long interview should take the form of a physical examination. Even after this the doubt may linger and it may be worth while getting another opinion. Anything is better than losing one's sleep. The following case is salutary.

Case 51 The patient, a woman of 30, was well-known to the doctors. She usually adopted a hostile attitude, more often than not presenting one of her children as a problem for which she required an exact diagnosis. The doctors were thus often compelled to undertake investigations which they considered unnecessary and even harmful to the children's well being. On one occasion she came to the surgery complaining of pain in the left side of the abdomen. Examination was normal. The patient was told she had colic and was given medicine containing an antispasmodic. She did not take kindly to this, remarking that colic was a diagnosis for horses. At the next interview arrangements were made for her to see a specialist. He carried out investigations, namely occult bloods, sigmoidoscopy and a barium enema, all of which were negative. A diagnosis was made of "irritable colon syndrome". The condition did not improve and the family doctor gave her a long psychiatric interview which was unrewarding and traumatic. She was referred back to the specialist who repeated the investigations, adding a full gastrointestinal survey. These were negative and the surgeon suggested a psychiatric opinion. This the patient refused. The surgeon's hand was finally forced and he admitted her to hospital for laparotomy. At operation the abdomen was found to be full of secondaries from a small carcinoma of the descending colon.

The long interview is usually the province of the psychiatrist. Family doctors may set aside time for this when short interviews have failed or the problem is obviously deep seated, such for example as severe grief reactions, marriage difficulties or sexual problems. The latter two I find unrewarding, probably because of my own lack of skill, so I usually refer these cases to someone better able to cope with them. I also rarely nowadays employ what people call a structured psychiatric interview. My long interviews with patients tend to be long chats or long periods of listening, in other words counselling rather than psychotherapy. I admire Cecily Saunders' expression "listening without technique" and this is what I try to do in most cases. However, it is wrong to listen without forming a relationship, as some analytical psychoanalysts do. This makes them into stuffed dummies and it is exceedingly boring to talk to a stuffed dummy. If the patient ceases to attend, the psychiatrist likes to think it is because he is "threatened" but the real reason is boredom and frustration. Balint, following the lead of Hippocrates, insisted that the doctor should offer himself as part of the treatment and the title of his well-known book "The Doctor, His Patient and the Illness" is a quotation from the Hippocratic Collection. Balint, more than anyone else, has made the long interview feasible for the family doctor and his colleagues have modified the technique to "six minutes for the patient".

For the psychiatrist the long interview is the standard procedure. For repeat visits the interview may be short, especially if the patient is under the National Health Service where pressures on time are severe. This can lead to disappointment because a patient who goes to hospital expects a long time with the psychiatrist and may not be satisfied with the five or ten minutes which he would accept as natural from his family doctor. It is however unavoidable. Patients seen privately will have a set time and so get their money's worth.

If a family doctor decides to send a patient to a psychiatrist his most important decision is to match the patient and the psychiatrist. The psychiatrist has no fore-knowledge so cannot select the patients he will be best able to help, so it is up to the family doctor. Failure to do this may be disastrous. A patient who needs a father may be landed with a husband, and so on. Also a patient who cannot bear to be exposed may have layer after layer of the onion stripped off him and I have seen this leading to tragedy. Another patient who needs to talk and talk may find himself wired-up to an ECT machine or so flattened with drugs that he cannot think. This, of course, is a picture of psychiatry at its worst. Most psychiatrists are broad-minded and have more experience than the family doctor in deciding what is best for the patient.

Case 52 The family doctor brought a psychiatrist to the home of a spinster of 35 who was suffering from depression of a rather indeterminate kind. She lived with her mother in a charming country cottage and was a well educated girl of strict moral upbringing. The two doctors were received in the drawing room with a tea tray on which were small sandwiches and cakes. After the introduction there was an embarrassed silence. The psychiatrist allowed this to go on for about two minutes, then said, "Why is it you are embarrassed to be in the same room as two men?".

This was a disastrous remark and did a lot of harm. Yet the psychiatrist was a capable and experienced doctor of the analytical type, very good at his job. The fault lay with the family doctor because he had brought the wrong psychiatrist to that particular house.

The third form of treatment, physical therapy, has its dangers too. Drugs should only be given after at least a preliminary discussion with the patient. The doctor should not reach for his prescription pad as soon as the patient admits to being worried. If I decide a patient has an anxiety state I usually prescribe tranquillisers for between a fortnight and a month. After this withdrawal becomes more difficult. Sleeping tablets I avoid if possible but there are a limited number of patients in whom insomnia is an entity. It may not be associated with anxiety symptoms and requires treatment because it is self-perpetuating and extremely disabling. Patients have told me that they "ache with fatigue" and I have experienced this myself after a night up. It seems almost a biochemical state and a few nights' good sleep may put it right.

Many conditions of course require long term treatment, months, years or forever. Some types of endogenous depression and schizophrenia have the feel of a physical rather than a mental illness and must be treated on these lines. Psychotherapy is anyway impossible because of lack of communication. It is these patients who often benefit from electroconvulsive therapy. Later they should be given help and encouragement in adjusting to a world from which they have temporarily withdrawn. Some patients need a permanent tiny dose of drugs, perhaps chlorpromazine for a schizophrenic or imipramine for a depressed patient.

There is a difference of opinion between psychiatrists and family doctors in the use of drugs. The psychiatrist tends to start with a big dose, and in my experience patients rarely take more than a few tablets because they feel so ill, unless of course they are in a mental hospital and have no choice. The family doctor usually starts on a small dose and works it up if necessary. This I find far more effective although my psychiatrist friends laugh if I tell them I have put a patient on imipramine 10 mgm three times a day, or amitryptilene 25 mgm at night. It seems to work for my patients.

Some physically orientated doctors become addicted to drugs. I do not mean by this that they slip off to the bathroom with an ampoule of heroin. I mean they become addicted to giving drugs to their patients. I have often seen patients on five or six different tranquillisers of which perhaps four are almost identical chemically. It is difficult to understand the logic of this. Sometimes it is just carelessness. A drug is added to the bottom of the list without removing the one from the top.

Many patients, quite rightly, prefer to do without tablets. I treated one girl of 25 with clomipramine (Anafranil) for depression. After a fortnight I asked her how she was. She replied, "Oh, I stopped taking the tablets. I felt better on them but I would rather be myself, thank you very much."

So I have described the three types of treatment for mental illness, an oversimplification but a useful oversimplification. Each is effective for the right patient and each has its dangers. Because I have stressed the dangers it does not mean I am an anti-psychiatrist – far from it. Psychiatrists are specialists and, like surgeons, are essential for the selected few, but the ordinary mortal may do better with help of a more simple kind. No-one wants their appendix removed unless it is the cause of the abdominal pain and no-one wants the onion layers peeled off if these are a useful form of protection. Those who talk of "their psychoanalyst" as they talk of their hairdresser have already become entangled in a net from which they may not be able to escape. They may not want to.

When one hears of a patient attending regular psychoanalytic sessions for seventeen years one wonders what has been attained. The answer is an expert psychoanalytical patient. He is an expert in a limited field and quite possibly more remote from the outside world than he had been seventeen years previously.

Also less happy. There is a paradox here. The saying "know thyself" is often quoted. There is another saying, by Hazlitt, "We never do anything well till we cease to think about the manner of doing it". This applies to how one lives one's life.

The aspect of psychiatry which especially interested Hippocrates was dream interpretation. All cultures are interested in dreams. Priests and seers have made their reputations on dream divination. In the Bible Joseph was so successful at this that he was taken from prison – where he had been incarcerated after an unfortunate affair with Potiphar's wife – and became the leading industrialist in Egypt. "Behold the dreamer", his brothers had said sarcastically, but it certainly paid dividends for Joseph.

Recently Freud stirred up the pool but now the water is settling, it seems that Freud's dream interpretations were no more accurate than those of Hippocrates, who also made lists of the symbolic meaning of objects.

4.447 *Crossing rivers, enemy soldiers and strange monsters indicate disease or madness.*

I hope Freud knew the following passage by heart:

4.421 *Dreams have a strong influence on all things. When the body is awake the spirit is its servant. The spirit is never her own mistress but divides her favours amongst hearing, sight, touch, walking, and all activities of the body. But when the body is asleep the spirit administers her own household and has perception of all things, sees what is visible, hears what is audible, walks, touches, feels pain, ponders. The spirit takes over the functions of the body during sleep and anyone who can interpret these acts know a great part of wisdom.*

Let us simplify the matter of dreams. Each of us sometimes wakes up feeling sublimely happy and if we are lucky can recall the dream which has been so fulfilling. Similarly we may wake up weighed down by a lump of misery and may recall this too. Often the dreams have obvious connections with everyday life or have easily interpreted symbolism. Beyond this we or the psychiatrist can start hunting for inner meanings, be it sloshing about in amniotic fluid or deciding we hate our parents or are in love with our secretaries. These interpretations cannot be proved true or untrue and the importance lies in the way we feel we should interpret the dream rather than any inherent sacrosanct meaning in the dream itself. That is why other people helping us interpret dreams can be so dangerous. It is a great big jolly game but in most games people can get hurt, especially if the rules are laid down at the whim of one person, Freud for example.

11

The Art, Philosophy and Religion

1.53 *Some physicians and philosophers consider that no-one can understand medicine unless they know what Man is. Unless a doctor learns this he cannot treat his patients correctly. He must be a philosopher and must understand the origins and meaning of mankind and how he evolved.*

I hold the opposite view, that the writings of physicians and philosophers about Nature have no more bearing on medicine than they do on painting. I also hold that knowledge of man's nature can be acquired from practical medicine and no other source — by this I mean what man is, how and why he is made and so on. I think a doctor must be at pains to find out the relationship of man to his environment, especially his food and drink, otherwise he cannot practice properly. To give an example he will learn from experience that "undiluted wine drunk in large quantities will produce a foreseeable effect on man".

This important passage appears at first reading to be a negation of much of what has been written in this book. It is something of a paradox. What Hippocrates is in fact saying is that we should start with man as he is and first relate him to his environment. This in turn will lead to a study of the environment itself, which will bring us to concepts of Nature. From there we take the ever winding path upwards to philosophy and religion. To Hippocrates it was a question of where we start and he believed that we should begin at the bottom and work upwards. He is not denying the value of philosophy but putting it in its right place. In other words he is saying, "The proper study of mankind is man". The example he gives about drinking wine may appear trite but it is an easily observed phenomenon. From this phenomenon it is permissible to build a theory of how the mind and nervous system works. This was just what Hughlings Jackson did. His ideas were developed in Sherrington's "Integrative Action of the Nervous System" which in turn led to the concept of relationships and Gestalts and so on up the winding stairway, which we will try to follow in this chapter.

1.35 *I want to return to those who conduct their researches in the art in the new way, building on a postulate.*

Hippocrates was fighting for the survival and development of science in medicine, that is to say a system based on observation. A postulate usually implies starting halfway up the stairs and this is something Hippocrates condemned. It is unfortunate that he had to fight this battle because, although he repeatedly said just the opposite, it contributed to the schism between medicine as a science and art, which we have today. He concentrated on science and the more practical aspects of the art. The rest he could leave to the dramatists and philosophers of which there was no shortage. That is why I have suggested Euripides as his alter ego; otherwise the picture is incomplete. In some ways Hippocrates is comparable to St. Paul, who launched Christianity on the world. St. Paul had to be dogmatic and he introduced distortions of Christ's teaching which still cause alarm and despondency. However he had little choice in the matter. Like Hippocrates with science, so St. Paul with Christianity. He had to get it off the ground.

1.127 *I, too, think these diseases are divine and so are all others, no one being more divine or natural than another; all are alike and*

> *all are divine. Each has its own nature and no disease arises without a natural cause.*

This is similar to a passage previously quoted. To Hippocrates there was no difference between what was divine and what was not divine. The distinction was meaningless. However it must be remembered that in more recent times anything which could not be explained scientifically was considered the work of God, the two being separate. Even Newton felt this way. He explained the rotation of the earth round the sun by his theory of gravity but considered the rotation of the earth round its own axis to be an act of God. The very expression "God knows!" implies that man does not know and it is not worth his while trying to find out. Unfortunately as science grows God diminishes, a ridiculous state of affairs suggesting that God will ultimately be squeezed out of existence.

People ask today, "Is there a God?" and books, radio and television try to give an answer. To Hippocrates this would have been a non-question. Of course there is a God. Of course there is not a God. I think time will show that Hippocrates was right. One of the characteristics of mankind, primitive or sophisticated, is a sensibility to what one might call a divine pattern, although there are many other words which could be used in its place equally well – Roget's Thesaurus gives a selection of over two hundred. We all have this sensibility although it can be diverted or partially suppressed. The real question that should be asked is, "In what way should we develop this sensibility?" To ask someone, "Is there a God?" is unfair. It implies he should give a yes or no answer in the same way as if we asked him, "Do you like bananas?" In some ways the Greeks were more sensible than we are.

1.355 *Life is a force in living creatures and their parts. It is also a force in all things, animate or inanimate.*

This force was personified by the Greeks in earlier times. Every stream had its nymph, every tree its dryad. The moon was a goddess, the constellations immortals. There was a spirit in all objects.

It is to the credit of the Greeks that they were able to hold on to these symbolic ideas alongside their development of scientific thinking. We seem unable to do this. The beauty of something is intrinsic and not related to our knowledge of how it works or to what extent we can analyse it. If the moon makes us think of Artemis (Diana) hunting the night skies this is a valid concept and nothing to do with the fact that astronauts have chipped bits of rock off its surface and brought them back to earth. The two ideas can live alongside each other – the romantic and the intellectual – with neither diminishing the value of the other. Unfortunately due to historical accident and a considerable element of bigotry on both sides the two are now looked upon as hated rivals. This is unnecessary because they deal with different aspects of the same thing and can even enhance each other if the mind is trained to switch from one to the other.

The Greek idea of gods was quite different from our own. For one thing there was a multitude of them, each representing an aspect of nature or life. A god of the same name in a different place would represent something different. Apollo of Delphi represented the sacred oracle, while Apollo Nomius was associated with lumpy faeces, as Hippocrates pointed out. This pantheism had its advantages. A single universal God cannot show indecision and cannot take sides. The Greek gods were nearly always indecisive and prejudiced. In World War I it is said there was genuine surprise when German and Allied troops talked with each other.

> "But God is on our side," one would say.
> "No, you're wrong. He's on our side," the other would reply.

Such a situation could not have occurred at Troy where the gods lined up like two football teams and when the game began used patently unfair tactics. Zeus was meant to be the referee but at moments of crisis he was almost invariably asleep or being seduced by one of the goddesses. He ranks as the worst referee of all time.

The reader may think I am making light of a serious matter but the way I have put it is only a slight exaggeration of what the Greeks thought. They had a tolerant, easy-going attitude to the gods. The poets from Homer onwards made good use of it. The question one asks is, "Were they gods at all?" They had little to do with moral laws. They were capricious, like the weather, and had to be appeased. Rarely were they worshipped or prayed to as the God of today. But at least they were acceptable and easy to understand because they were not much different from humans. This, however, led many Greeks to feel the need for a divine spirit beyond the gods. "She is more than a god", wrote Euripides of Aphrodite in one of his plays, suggesting paradoxically that the Greek gods were only divine on special occasions.

We, because of our place in history, tend to think of God as both remote and intimate. He creates a tension in us because we have to keep Him at arm's length although we would dearly like to chat with Him, as Don Camillo used to in his little village church. The compromise of course is to create God in the image of man and like the fish in Rupert Brookes' poem we are really rather stupid about it. To fish, God is a super-fish:

> "Immense, of fishy form and mind,
> Squamous, omnipotent, and kind;
> And under that Almighty Fin,
> The littlest fish may enter in."

The essence of Christianity is to bridge the gap by a concept called incarnation. Christ was both God and man but it is very difficult for anyone, apart from a saint, to understand this fully. If, like the Greeks, we reduce God to human form we have to think of a divine pattern beyond this form and hence we start fragmenting God. We should be honest enough to accept this and realise that any definition or interpretation of God is bound to be a failure although it may be a useful working premise. To think further is to become entangled in theology and lose sight of the Essence, as Hippocrates called it.

1.299 *I swear by Apollo Physician, by Asclepius, by Health, by Panacea and by all the gods and goddesses, making them my witness, that I will carry out, according to my ability and judgement, this oath and this indenture.*

This is how the scientifically minded Greeks swore their oath to maintain the ideals laid down by Hippocrates. We could not bring ourselves to do this and, sadly, some of us have nothing to swear by apart, perhaps, from the Secretary of State for Social Services or his equivalent in other countries outside the United Kingdom. However, we can take comfort from the fact that when the Greeks invoked Apollo, Asclepius (Aesculapius) and so on they were doing little more than appealing to the master physicians, albeit partly mythical, of a previous era. It is not unlike a British doctor swearing by "Hippocrates, Galen and the past presidents of the Royal Colleges".

2.287 *The physician who is a lover of wisdom is the equal of a god.*

If a professor qualifies automatically for divinity it does not say much for divinity. The truth is we are blinded by the beauty of Greek literature into thinking their religion was comparable with the great religions of today. In fact it was primitive. Their gods were at heart the gods of barbaric tribes. Mostly they came from the north, first a wave of predominantly female figures, nymphs and goddesses, who were set up locally, then a wave of predominantly male gods who had to take over the existing deities. Hence the stories of seduction in Greek myth. Apollo appeared to spend his time raping, or attempting to rape nymphs, and Zeus was not much better. He was not a figure of respect and Aristophanes in his play "The Clouds" was able to put forward the theory that rain was "Zeus pissing through a sieve". We cannot correlate this with the single God of today.

It was from Greek philosophy rather than Greek religion that we inherited some of our ideas of the pattern of divinity I have described. "In the beginning was the Word, and the Word was with God, and the Word was God." This, the opening lines of the Gospel according to St. John, is a concept of Greek philosophy, and when we think of philosophers we think of Socrates, who was a contemporary of Hippocrates.

Socrates was a religious man. He accepted the reality of a single divine force beyond the mythical gods and goddesses yet was himself a cause of division between mankind and divinity. We hear of him mainly through Plato's Dialogues, so we never know if it is Socrates or Plato we are listening to. Be that as it may, Socrates believed truth could be reached by reason alone. His trade was argument or dialectic. He, or one of his followers, would put forward a postulate and they would proceed to dissect, analyse and break it down. Nothing can be assumed. Ordinary conversation with Socrates must have been almost an impossibility and this so irritated the Athenians that they called him "the gadfly".

His methods were not those of Hippocrates. He was not quite one of those "who conduct their researches in the new way, building on postulates", because his way was to tear postulates to pieces. Hippocrates worked through observation, Socrates reasoning, and the formal scientist of today combines the two.

2.289 *The study of medicine weaves into the stuff of the mind knowledge of the gods.*

Does this mean that all doctors are religious or become religious? In a sense, yes. Because they have frequent contact with the inner thoughts of others, in particular their fears and sorrows, they have for very practical reasons to develop a philosophy. This is to help their patients as well as for their own survival. We use the expression "being philosophical about things" and this is exactly what a doctor has to be. If a patient dies or, even more, if the doctor has to tell, say, a wife that her husband is going to die, he cannot let it spoil his own life.

2.227 *There are some arts which cause a lot of stress to those that employ them but are of great benefit to mankind. Such an art is what the Greeks call the art of medicine. For a doctor sees terrible things, touches unpleasant things, and the misfor-*

tunes of others bring a harvest of sorrows that are peculiarly his own.

He must learn to experience and live with these sorrows. He may become hardened and be unable to share his patient's grief and anxieties, in which case he has not much to offer them. Or he may become too involved and cease to work efficiently as a doctor. The true professional is the doctor who can keep a balance between the two.

This necessitates philosophy and, for many, the difference between philosophy and religion nowadays is nominal. The traditionally religious will point out that the word "nominal" means in name only and that name is God; a choice has to be made. As I have already said, I believe this choice to be an artificial one and often a stumbling block between like-minded people. The word god has connotations that go back to the Greeks and beyond and are not always relevant today. As Hippocrates said, the word is not the same as the essence.

It is difficult to write about religion because each of us has his own view point. I am a practising Christian largely because I was brought up that way and because, with literature and music, Christianity expresses my sensibility to the "divine Pattern". I cannot claim that Christianity is nearer the truth than Islam, Buddhism or Hinduism because I have only read about these religions. I have not experienced them. To try to experience them all would make one into a sort of religious dilettante and probably diminish one's sensibility, because one would be studying religion as a subject.

As a doctor I have to take a very practical line and, to modify once again Nelson's signal before Trafalgar, I would say that in any situation if in doubt one cannot go far wrong if one does what Christ would have done. This will have to do for the time being.

4.423 *Prayer is good but while calling on the gods a man should lend a hand.*

These are memorable words. There are doctors, but they must

be very few nowadays, who feel they do signal service for their individual patients by praying on their behalf. The doctor is an intermediary but not an active intermediary. There are, however, very many doctors who believe that their contact with the divine pattern, be it by prayer to God or a deepening of their sensibility by any other means, makes them a much more efficient instrument of healing. If I happen to pick up a Mozart symphony on the car radio on my way to the surgery my patients will benefit enormously. I will be quite kind to the first two or three. If, however, it is Bartok or, worse still, a materialistic news item of an unpleasant nature, their reception will not be nearly so good.

A doctor of any religious faith, who understands and practises prayer in a way I cannot, would receive enormous power if he meditated for ten minutes before each clinic or, if he was a surgeon, before each operating session – but only if he carried in his mind the dictum of Hippocrates which we are considering. Otherwise the contrast between the peace of contact with divinity and practical medicine is too traumatic and can be harmful. "Why is it", the nurses on a particular ward used to say, "that Sister is always in such a bad temper when she's been to early morning Communion?" The answer was that she was unwilling to "lend a hand" and God was not prepared to write her ward reports or deal with fractious patients or staff on her behalf.

However, the true impact of religion on the doctor is his realisation of the importance of the patient. Much of what I said in the previous chapters about literature is relevant to religion but more so, because there is no doubt in my own mind that true religion is the greatest development of sensibility there can be. Unfortunately in Western culture it is now rare, although I suppose but do not know from personal experience that in Eastern religions it is far more common and acceptable.

It is customary for devout Buddhists as they get old to spend many hours a day studying their scriptures to prepare themselves for death. The passage between life and death is gradual. If a "senior citizen" in Britain did this he would be considered morbid and would find himself being taken to a Derby and Joan

Club every Tuesday and Friday, or even be put on antidepressants. A doctor should have enough sensibility to realise that elderly patients sometimes have a profound need of this sort and they should not be jollied out of it. This is not in the medical curriculum, but death is part of the doctor's trade and he should understand it. Preparation for death is, I believe, an essential part of life and is beneficial unless it is morbid – like the poet Donne sleeping in a shroud, or uneconomic – like the Pharoahs building pyramids.

4.249 *Men do not understand how to see the invisible through the visible. They do not realise the arts they employ are reflections of their own natures. For all things are like and unlike, compatible and incompatible, communicating and non-communicating, intelligent and without intelligence. Each is a paradox.*

This passage is difficult to interpret. It presumably means that men find it hard to understand anything which is not made available to them through their own sense organs. It is the development of comprehension beyond the immediate sensations that differentiates man from other animals. He is aware of awareness. This sensibility, according to Teilhard de Chardin in his "Phenomenon of Man", will continue to evolve, not by any change or increase in the cells of the cerebral cortex but by psychosocial evolution which has taken over from Darwinian type evolution and is much swifter. No-one knows how far this sensibility may develop. It could be that there will be some kind of break-through in the future and people will talk of the Spiritual Revolution as they now talk of the Technological, Industrial and Agricultural Revolutions.

"The arts they employ being the reflections of their own nature" implies what has been said repeatedly in the book. Man creates what he perceives far more than he realises and his actions are reflections of himself. The doctor who thinks he is being objective is probably deceiving himself because he cannot exclude his own nature from a situation in which he is involved. As Hippocrates and Balint after him have said, the art of medicine consists of the doctor, the patient and his illness. The doctor cannot be excluded from this trio.

4.249 *Man arranges things by custom but the natural order is arranged by the gods. What man arranges is never constant, whether right or wrong, but what the gods arrange is right forever.*

This indicates a belief in a universal moral law. The philosopher Kant said, "Two things fill the mind with ever-increasing wonder and awe, the more often and the more intensely the mind of thought is drawn to them: the starry heavens above me and the moral law within me."

This moral law is subject to interpretation and distortion as we well know from events of the past and of our own times. It is fashionable nowadays to deny the existence of a moral law. The fresh air of existentialism has proved to be an icy blast, but with luck a thaw is on the way. Heavy-handed morality is equally chilling but there can be a compromise.

A doctor of today is expected to exhibit a high moral code but, paradoxically, he must have an existential attitude towards his patients. He is split two ways and if he has different codes for his private and public life it means he is split three ways. This is a very difficult situation to tolerate and the doctor must come to terms with it.

1.345 *The beginning of all things is one and the end of all things is one and the end and the beginning are the same.*

It is easy to read universal concepts into the words of Hippocrates and, in context, this passage may mean little more than a comment on the digestive tract. However it simulates so closely the opening lines of one of the poems in T. S. Eliot's "Four Quartets" that I choose to give it a wider interpretation.

> "What we call the beginning is often the end
> And to make an end is to make a beginning.
> The end is where we start from."

"Four Quartets" is, amongst other things, a group of poems about Time. For ages the dimensions of Time and Space have been looked upon as the clue to the relationship between the visible and invisible. We use expressions like "timeless", "eternal" which means far more than going on forever, and we talk of "beyond space and time", although the use of the preposition "beyond" implies a further dimension by which times and space can be measured.

J. W. Dunne in his book "An Experiment with Time" worked out a mathematical explanation of this which I cannot pretend to understand. He symbolised the extended human mind, if we may call it that, as an artist painting a picture who is himself being painted by another artist. He is being painted by a third artist and so it goes on through an infinite series of dimensions. Each artist can see the ones below him in the scale but he cannot see himself nor the artists above him, although he may be aware of their existence. Our human brain copes up to the fourth artist, as it were, seeing the picture (time) and the three other artists (space) below us.

This is an interpretation of what Hippocrates wrote:

4.429 *Men do not understand how to see the invisible through the visible.*

And Socrates said, "If we are to know anything absolutely we must be free from the body and behold the actual realities with the eye of the soul."

As I see it, the cerebral cortex is, through the sense organs, in contact with a four dimensional world which it can interpret and measure. The divine, God, the pattern, quality, essence, or whatever you wish to call it cannot be understood or measured because it is in the series but on the wrong side. The artist cannot see the artist who is painting him. As a fourteenth-century monk put it, there is a "cloud of unknowing" which we cannot pierce.

This to me is a startlingly obvious truth. It is also supported by common sense. If I play a game of chess the chessmen have a three dimensional existence, two of space, one of time. If they could think they would not be aware of me, a sort of Aeschylian divine power from a higher dimension, who decrees that bishops move diagonally and knights three spaces forward and one to the side. People have in fact devised a "four dimensional" form of chess which is very difficult for the player to grasp. A five dimensional game is theoretically possible but beyond human comprehension.

Similarly when we watch television we are seeing a three dimensional world in action, two of space and one of time, although by various optical illusions we make it a four dimensional Gestalt. If we peer at the back of the set there is no doubt that one of the dimensions has gone missing. Life on the television screen is independent of our own. They cannot see us but we can see them. Nor, in this instance, can we alter what is taking place apart from switching the set off or going through a vastly complex procedure of 'phoning the programme controller of the B.B.C.

If this is accepted as a general truth, without necessarily any complex mathematics, everything begins to fall into place. It is more profitable to think of God as those dimensions beyond the measurable perception of our cerebral cortex but of which we are partially aware through sensibility rather than sense. It is helpful for many people to personalise this because it brings Him within our range of understanding.

Furthermore we can understand death. As Hippocrates said,

2.179 *The brain . . . acts as the interpreter of the phenomena of the outside world. . . . The brain is the messenger of consciousness.*

It is illogical to think that, when the brain is dead and the cortical cells decayed, thoughts go ticking on all by themselves. An after life is impossible, if by "after" we mean something later in the dimension of time we understand. However, the dead person's life exists in the further series of dimensions. It has to. I can, as an analogy, draw a line, as at the top of the opposite page, and postulate that it represents a person's life in two dimensions, one of space and one of time. He is born at the beginning of the line and dies at the end. He has ceased to be, and one can even see the space where he ought to be. But the line is still there and we in our superior position of an artist of the fourth dimension can look at it for as long as we want.

This brings us the salubrious thought that everything we say or do survives for ever. In fact everything that has ever happened survives for ever. We do not have to look much further for heaven and hell. Hell is the cruel remark we made ten years ago, heaven a moment of kindness or beauty long since forgotten. We spend eternity looking at our lives.

In Tolkien's "Lord of the Rings" the elf-queen, Galadriel, has a magic mirror, which is a basin of clear water. She says, "What you will see, if you leave the mirror free to work, I cannot tell. For it shows things that were, and things that are, and things that yet may be. But which it is that he sees, even the wisest cannot always tell. Do you wish to look?"

No, we do not wish to look, not at the moment, because, as T. S. Eliot put it:

> ". . . to apprehend
> The point of intersection of the timeless
> With time, is an occupation for the saint."

We must stop sloshing about in metaphysics and return to the practical day to day work of the doctor. I hope what I have written has helped to clear the path. It is not my intention to expound any particular religion or philosophy but I have tried to show that if the reader accepts in approximation what has been said he will be able to appreciate his own and other's sensibility to the divine pattern in whatever form it takes, and conclude it is as real, or more real, than the world of Newtonian physics – or Einstein's physics if he can understand it. This has several practical applications in his relationship to the patient.

First, he must be prepared to pay attention to this sensibility if the occasion demands it.

Second, he must not despise the form this sensibility takes if it appears illogical or different from his own probably very personal ideas. I have long ceased arguing with Mormons, Jehovah's Witnesses, extreme Catholics or Fundamentalists and believers in faiths or philosophies which I do not understand. What is good enough for the patient is good enough for me and if they choose a particular basis for their life, unless it is obviously evil, I will go along with them. A patient I once saw told me she was a witch, and having made sure she did not use her "powers" to harm people, I found her attitudes helpful in relation to her illness.

Third, life has a reality far greater than apears on the surface, so every patient is important. The trivial or ugly should be seen in this light.

Fourth, death can be conceived as an illusion because everything is for ever. Hence if the dying person or the bereaved find comfort in this concept or "hope to meet their loved ones in another world" they have reason on their side. It is not just a sentimental whim which, under the circumstances, is quite natural. A doctor need not have faith himself in order to accept the patient's faith. A doctor who is, say, a Christian may be formalising the ideas of a doctor who is, say, a humanist or atheist. There need be no conflict of ideas.

And fifth . . .

1.319 *For where there is love of man there is love of the art. For some patients though conscious that their condition is perilous recover their health simply through their contentment with the goodness of the physician. And it is good to look after the sick, to make them well, to care for the healthy, to keep them well, but also to care for one's own self so as to do what is right.*

Epilogue: The Paradox of the Art

1.359 *Blood is liquid and blood is solid. Liquid blood is good, liquid blood is bad. Solid blood is good, solid blood is bad. All things are good or bad relatively. The way up, the way down.*

The Greeks loved paradox. By this one means a statement which contains opposites, both of which are true in part. The most famous exponent of the art of paradox was the Oracle at Delphi, which was believed to be the centre of the world, the omphalos or tummy-button. The Oracle would make a paradoxical statement leaving the recipient to discover the truth as it applied to himself. Many will remember the story of Croesus who decided to attack the Persian Empire and sent to the Oracle at Delphi for its opinion. He was told that if he went to war he would destroy a mighty empire. He accordingly carried out his plans, which he would have done anyway. Unfortunately it was his own empire that was destroyed.

A similar paradoxical answer was given to the Athenians when they were about to fight the Persians. They were told their salvation would lie in their "wooden walls", which could mean either the walls of the Acropolis or their fleet of wooden ships. They decided on the latter and in this case the decision was the correct one.

The Delphic Oracle fell into disrepute over the Greek–Persian wars. It appeared so certain that Xerxes would win that the Oracle chanced its arm and made a non-paradoxical statement, one of the rare occasions when its political acumen was faulty. As everyone knows, the Persian army annihilated a detachment of Spartans at Thermopylae but later their fleet was heavily defeated at Salamis.

> "A King sate on the rocky brow
> Which looks o'er sea-born Salamis;
> And ships, by thousands, lay below,
> And men in nations; – all were his!
> He counted them at break of day –
> And when the sun set where were they?"

The Athenian "wooden walls" had done their work and after other defeats the Persians were finally routed at Plataea. The Delphic Oracle was not popular, especially since its pessimistic verdict had helped some Greek states decide to fight on the side of the Persians.

Oracular statements are not often made nowadays but it is a valuable weapon in the doctor's armament once he has learnt the art. It implies making a statement which is neither indefinite nor untrue but gives the patient a choice of interpretation. It is especially relevant to situations where the patient has cancer or is likely to die. Indecision or obscurity increases the patient's anxiety but if the doctor states that salvation lies, as it were, in the "wooden walls" the patient can decide what the wooden walls are. He may, for example, interpret the doctor's statement as meaning he has not got cancer; or he has got cancer but he will be all right; or that he is going to die of cancer but it is nothing to fear.

The art of medicine itself is a paradox because for each positive statement there is usually the converse which in its own context is equally true. This book, as the reader will have noted, is full of paradoxes or, if he is less kind, he will call it confusion. This is because, if Hippocrates is right and medicine is a balance of opposites, these opposites must be stated and the reader must make his choice. As with the Delphic Oracle he chooses what is right for him.

For example it is made clear that a doctor, to be complete, must form strong personal attachments to patients when the need arises but at the same time he must avoid attachments which will be harmful both to himself and the patients. He must peel off many layers of the onion if he can thereby discover the patient's illness. Yet peeling onions is a destructive process in itself and the oracle will not tell him if the mighty empire he will destroy is the illness or the patient, or possibly even himself.

The doctor nowadays has effective methods of treatment for most diseases yet anything that is effective is also harmful, so the better his treatment the more likely it is to harm the patient. He is forever creating and destroying, and conversely if he does not make mistakes he is not likely to help his patients very much.

He is exhorted to identify diseases in the early stages, in particular by the use of screening techniques, yet screening creates illness as well as revealing it. The wider he casts his net the more red herrings he will catch. Similarly the patient is advised to visit his doctor early before the disease has developed and at the same time is told he must not waste the doctor's time with trivial matters.

The patient expects to be given medicine as a token of the doctor's interest and care, then is told that he should not use the doctor as a purveyor of tablets but buy them himself from the chemist or that he shouldn't have medicine at all. On the other hand the doctor is expected to let Nature cure the disease, especially an infective illness, if he thinks this is likely to happen, but is put under pressure to prescribe an antibiotic.

The doctor is encouraged, as a discipline, to make a diagnosis in all illness yet he is also taught that a diagnosis is often illusory, an escape for himself, and he should really be seeking the answer to a problem. He should think of the patient not the disease, yet if he does that he misses the disease, while if he thinks of the disease he forgets the patient. Time is his ally and will give him the answer, yet time is his enemy and he must not depend on it. He is forever short of time but the more time he has the shorter it seems. Somehow he must pick his way through this mire of opposites.

In a wider field he must protect the patient from the environment and improve the environment for the patient, yet if there is no conflict between man and his environment lethargy sets in and illness is created. If there is conflict stress occurs and the patient will need help to overcome it.

The doctor, as a scientist, must be objective. He must observe each situation as a new entity but he has to rely on the experience and knowledge handed to him by others, although what is considered right today will be obsolete or even wrong tomorrow. If he is completely objective his perception of the patient will be arid and futile, so he has to rely on imagination and fantasy to complete the picture. If he does this he is seeking self-safisfaction and may distort the truth. He must be precise but imaginative in his speech and writing yet precision is close to technical terminology and the imaginative expression which "catches on" becomes jargon. He must try to estimate the quality of his work although quality is, by definition, immeasurable. To understand something he must take it to pieces, but if he fails to put it together again he will lose the very thing he is trying to understand.

The patient should be self-reliant yet the doctor demands dependence from the patient in order to function as a doctor. The doctor should behave naturally yet he must forever play roles to suit the patient and he expects the patient to play roles to suit him. He should not, however, act his part so well as to unduly influence the patient but if he acts badly the play becomes a farce. He must withhold his personality but if he does he becomes a "hollow man" and the patient cannot form a relationship with him. He must analyse his patient's psychological problems yet analysis itself alters both the problem and the relationship; and if he analyses his own attitudes and method of working he destroys his natural style and his intimacy with the patient. He has to be a friend and a doctor but the two do not mix.

In the field of ethics the doctor must have a strict moral code but is not allowed to enforce it on the patient. He must school himself to take part in matters he may find distasteful, such for example as termination of pregnancy, considering it, in the famous oxymoron of Sophocles' Antigone, "a holy crime". However strong his religious, philosophical or political beliefs he must not use these to influence his patients, yet without beliefs he will find his work unsupportable. He must consider his job a vocation, even if he does not call it that, yet he has to earn his living and ensure he has adequate reward for his work.

He must compete with his colleagues but not be jealous of them or belittle them. As a teacher he must not harm his pupils, but only by harming them at times can he teach them. Similarly to learn himself he must expect to be hurt but must not allow his carefully nurtured defences to be penetrated. Discussion without conflict is valueless, yet conflict makes nonsense of discussion.

He must have sensibility towards his patient and be aware of sensibility to some sort of divine pattern but seldom or never speak of it. If he is of a "religious" turn of mind and believes that God created man in his own image he must also understand that man created God in his own image. He has a desire to pierce the "cloud of unknowing" but this is by definition impenetrable because his cerebral cortex is not up to it. He cannot succeed, but to keep on trying is success. He must think about the present yet be ready for the future. He should not dwell on the idea of death but should prepare his patients and himself for death.

This then is the Art of Medicine. We start with the unbiased observation of Hippocrates, create a pattern with the accumulated experience of doctors throughout the ages, interpret it with science and psychology, make it alive with sensibility to humanity, the arts, divinity or what you will. All these are in a state of tension, but the tension, if balanced, is harmony. I do not believe the Art has been forgotten but this could well happen if we ignore the message of Hippocrates, or fail to put it into practice.

There are many ways to the art of medicine and each doctor must choose the best one for himself. I have, in this book, chosen one particular way but I hope it will not be set up to the exclusion of other ways. Observation, science, psychology, creativeness, sensibility – each is a valid approach. All I have tried to do, with the help of Hippocrates and in the words of Newton, is to pick up a few bright pebbles from the seashore because they happen to please me.

The Oath – Modern Interpretation

1.299 *I swear by everything that is sacred to me that I will obey this oath to the best of my ability and judgement.*

I will respect my teacher as I would my parents and will ensure he is adequately rewarded and will pass on his teaching to others of my profession.

I will use treatment to help the sick to the best of my ability and judgement, but never to do them harm.

I will not administer harmful substances to anyone if asked to do so, nor will I suggest such an action.

I will not procure abortion in a woman.

I will keep my personal life and my work pure and upright.

I will undertake no act which I am not adequately trained to perform but will leave it to those who are expert.

Whenever I enter a house I will enter to help the sick.

I will abstain from all intentional wrong-doing and harm and will not abuse the privilege of examining the bodies of men or women, rich or poor.

I will keep secret anything I shall see or hear in the course of my professional duties and in everyday life which should not be told to other people.

If I carry out this oath I hope to gain a good reputation as a doctor and a person. If I fail to carry it out I will expect to get what I deserve.

The Oath – Original Version

1.299 *I swear by Apollo Physician, by Asclepius, by Health, by Panacea and by all gods and goddesses, making them my witnesses, that I will carry out, according to my ability and judgement, this oath and this indenture.*

To hold my teacher in this art equal to my own parents; to make him partner of my livelihood; when he is in need of money to share mine with him; to consider his family as my own brothers, and to teach them this art, if they want to learn it without fee or indenture; to impart precept, oral instruction, and all other instruction to my own sons, the sons of my teacher, and to indentured pupils who have taken the physician's oath, but to nobody else.

I will use treatment to help the sick according to my ability and judgement, but never with a view to injury or wrong-doing. Neither will I administer a poison to anybody when asked to do so, nor will I suggest such a course. Similarly I will not give to a woman a pessary to cause abortion. But I will keep pure and holy both my life and my art.

I will not use the knife, not even, verily, on sufferers from stone, but I will give place to such as are craftsmen therein.

Into whatsoever houses I enter, I will enter to help the sick, and I will abstain from all intentional wrong-doing and harm, especially from abusing the bodies of man or woman, bond or free.

And whatsoever I shall see or hear in the course of my profession, as well as outside my profession in my intercourse with men, if it be what should not be published abroad, I will never divulge, holding such things to be holy secrets. Now if I carry out this oath and break it not, may I gain forever reputation among all men for my life and for my art; but if I transgress it and forswear myself, may the opposite befall me.

Bibliography

The first part of this bibliography is for students of Hippocrates. The second part is an assortment of books and articles consisting of those I have consulted before writing this book, or to which reference has been made; those I have happened to come across while writing and have found helpful.

The list could of course be multiplied ten times. The reader is referred to an excellent biography of general practice in J. L. Stevens' Butterworth Gold Medal Essay (see below) and to any local library where he will find many good books on Greek culture.

Part 1 Hippocrates

Books

CHADWICK, J. and MANN, W. N., *The medical works of Hippocrates.* Blackwell. Oxford. 1950.

CHADWICK, J. and MANN, W. N., *Hippocratic Writings.* Edited by G. E. R. Lloyd. Penguin. Harmondsworth. 1978.

JONES, W. H. S., *Hippocrates.* Loeb Classical Library. Heinemann. London.

Vol. 1, 1923. Reprinted 1957.

Vol. 2, 1923. Reprinted 1959.

Vol. 4, 1931. Reprinted 1959.

LEVINE, EDWIN B., *Hippocrates.* World authors series No. 165. Twayne. New York.

WITHINGTON, E. T., *Hippocrates.* Loeb Classical Library. Heinemann. London.

Vol. 3, 1928. Reprinted 1959.

Articles

CHARLTON, M. H., *Hippocrates and Asklepios: rise and fall of ancient scientific neurology*. N.Y. State J. Med. **75**(i): 117, 9th Jan 1975.

CLARKE, E., *Apoplexy in the Hippocratic writings*. Bull. Hist. Med. **37**: 301 14 July–Aug 1963.

DUBOS, R., *Hippocrates in modern dress*. Perspect. Biol. Med. **9**: 175–88 Winter 1966.

FINLEY, J. H. Junr., *Hippocrates and classic Greece*. Bull. John Hopkins Hosp. **110**: 23–27 Jan 1962.

KATZ, A. M., *Hippocrates and the plane tree on the island of Cos*. Arch. Intern. Med. **104**: 653–7. October 1959.

MEERLOO, J. A., *Hippocrates and the methodical art of clinical thinking*. Int. Rec. Med. **173**: 643–50, October 1960.

MICHLER, M., *Medical ethics in Hippocratic bone surgery*. Bull. Hist. Med. **42**: 297–311. July–August 1968.

PENFIELD, W., *Hippocrates' environment and times, fact and fiction*. Clin. Neurosurg. (Baltimore) **4**: 11–20. 1956 (1957).

RODDIS, L., *From the case books of Hippocrates. Case reports for diagnosis*. Milit. Med. **129**: 143–4, Feb 1964.

SIEGEL, R. E., *Clinical observation in Hippocrates*. J. Mount Sinai Hosp. NY. **31**: 283–285 July–Aug 1964.

SIEGEL, R. E., *Epidemics and infectious diseases at the time of Hippocrates*. Gesnerus **17**: 77–98. 1960.

WILLIAMS, C. H., *Hippocrates: medical giant in the saga of men*. Md. State Med. J. **22**: 56–8. May 1973.

WILLIS, C. D., *Hippocrates revisited*. Bulletin. Hist. Med. (Baltimore) **32**: (6) 569–70 Nov–Dec 1958.

Part 2 General

AGNEW, L. R. C., *Humanism in medicine*. Lancet 2.596. 1977.

ANON, *The Cloud of Unknowing*. John M. Watkins. London. 1950.

ASHER, R., *Talking Sense*. Pitman Medical. Tunbridge Wells. 1972.

BALINT, E. and NORELL, J. S., *Six minutes for the patient: Interactions in General Practice Consultation*. Tavistock. London. 1973.

BALINT, M., *The Doctor, His Patient and the Illness*. Pitman Medical, Tunbridge Wells. 1968.

BARTLETT, SIR FREDERIC, *Remembering: Study in Experimental and Social Psychology*. Cambridge University Press. 1967.

BERNE, E., *Games People Play: Psychology of Human Relationships*. Deutsch. London. 1966.

BLACK, D., *Cui bono*. BMJ. 1977. 2.1109.

BOYERS, R. (Editor), *Laing and Anti-psychiatry*. Penguin. Harmondsworth. 1972.

BROWNE, K. and FREELING, P., *The Doctor—Patient Relationship*. Churchill Livingstone. London. 1976.

BURN, A. R., *The Pelican History of Greece*. Penguin. Harmondsworth. 1970.

BYRNE, P. DE LONG, *Doctors Talking to Patients*. H.M.S.O. 1976.

CHARDIN, P. TEILHARD DE, *The Phenomenon of Man*. Collins. London. 1959.

COULSON, C. A., *Science and Christian Belief*. O.U.P. 1955.

DAVIES, H., *Modern Medicine: a doctor's dissent*. Abelard. London. 1977.

DUNNE, J. W., *An Experiment with Time*. Faber and Faber. London. 1939.

DUNNE, J. W., *Nothing Dies*. Faber and Faber. London. 1950.

DURANT, W., *The Story of Philosophy*. Benn. London. 1947.

ELIOT, T. S., *Four Quartets*. Faber and Faber. London. 1944.

ELLIOTT-BINNS, C. P., *Personal View*. B.M.J. 1977. **2**: 314.

ELLIOTT-BINNS, C. P., *An Analysis of Lay Medicine*. J. Royal Coll. Gen. Pract. 1973. **23**: 255.

ELLIOTT-BINNS, C. P., HOOKER, A. N. and WILLIS, A. W., *Seeing two doctors at once in general practice*. J. Royal Coll. Gen. Pract. 1976. **26**: 684.

FARRINGTON, B., *Greek Science*. Penguin. Harmondsworth. 1944.

FERGUSON, J., *A Companion to Greek Tragedy*. University of Texas Press. Austin and London. 1972.

FORDHAM, FRIEDA, *An Introduction to Jung's Psychology*. Penguin. Harmondsworth. 1970.

FREEMAN, J. and BYRNE, P. S., *The Assessment of Vocational Training for General Practice*. Journal of the Royal College of General Practitioners. London. 1976.

FREUD, S., *The Psychopathology of Everyday Life*. Benn. London. 1960.

FRY, J. et al., *Self care: its place in the total health care system*. A report by an independent working party. London. 1973 (including bibliography).

FURLONG, MONICA, *The End of our Exploring*. Hodder. London. 1973.

"FYNN", *Mister God, This is Anna*. Collins. London. 1974.

GENERAL MEDICAL COUNCIL, *Professional Conduct and Discipline*. London. 1977.

GRAVES, R., *The Anger of Achilles*. Cassell. London. 1960.

GUARESCHI, G., *The Little World of Don Camillo*. Gollancz. London. 1951.

HUDSON, L., *Frames of Mind*. Methuen. London. 1968.

ILLICH, I., *Limits to Medicine*. Boyars. London. 1976.

JUNG, C. G., *Modern Man in Search of a Soul*. Routledge & Kegan Paul. London. 1933.

KITTO, H. D. F., *The Greeks*. Penguin. Harmondsworth. 1969.

KOESTLER, A., *The Act of Creation*. Hutchinson. London. 1969.

LAING, R. D., *The Divided Self*. Penguin. Harmondsworth. 1970.

LIVINGSTONE, SIR R. W. (Editor), *The Legacy of Greece*. Oxford University Press. 1921.

MADDEN, T., *Let 22,000 Flowers Bloom*. World Medicine 12.24. 17–32. 1977.

MARSH, G. N., *Curing minor illness in general practice*. B.M.J. **2**: 1267. 1977.

MAUGHAM, W. S., *Ten Novels and Their Authors.* Heinemann. London. 1963.

MCKEOWN, T., *The Role of Medicine*. Nuffield Provincial Hospital Trust. London. 1976.

MEDAWAR, P. B., *The Art of the Soluble: Creativity and Originality in Science.* Methuen. London. 1967.

MORRIS, D., *The Naked Ape.* Cape. London. 1967.

MUNTHE, A., *The Story of San Michele*. Murray. London. 1929.

PAFFARD, M., *The Unattended Moment*. SCM. London. 1976.

PAYNE, R., *The Triumph of the Greeks.* Hamish Hamilton. London. 1964.

PIRSIG, R. M., *Zen and the Art of Motorcycle Maintenance.* Bodley Head. London. 1974.

POPPER, K. R., *Conjectures and Refutations: Growth of Scientific Knowledge.* Routledge & Kegan Paul. London. 1963.

POST, L. VAN DEN, *Jung and the Story of Our Time.* Hogarth. London. 1976.

RHODES, P., *The Value of Medicine*. Allen and Unwin. London. 1977.

RIEU, E. V. (Translator), Homer. *The Iliad.* Penguin. Harmondsworth. 1950.

ROBINSON, E. and SUMMERFIELD, G., *Clare.* Oxford University Press. 1966.

RYLE, J. A., *The Aims and Methods of Medical Science*. Cambridge University Press. 1935.

SCHUMACHER, E. F., *Small is Beautiful: Study of Economics as if People Mattered.* Blond and Briggs. London. 1973.

SOWERBY, P., *The Doctor, his Patient and the Illness; a Reappraisal*. J. Royal College General Practitioners. 1977. **27**: 583–589.

STEVENS, J. L., *Quality of Care in General Practice; can it be Assessed?* (Butterworth Gold Medal Essay 1976). J. Royal College General Practitioners 1977. **27**: 455–466.

TIBBLE, J. W. and ANNE, *John Clare. A Life* (revised). Michael Joseph. London. 1972.

TOLKIEN, J. R. R., *The Lord of the Rings*. Allen & Unwin. London. 1966.

URANG, G., *Shadows of Heaven*. SCM Press. London. 1971.

VELLACOTT, P. (Translator), *Euripides. Alcestis and Other Plays*. Penguin. Harmondsworth. 1970.

VERNON, M. D., *The Psychology of Perception*. Penguin. Harmondsworth. 1970.

VERNON, P. E. (Editor), *Creativity.* Penguin. Harmondsworth. 1970.

WARNER, R., *Athens at War*. Bodley Head. London. 1970.

WARNER, R. (Translator), *Three Great Plays of Euripides*. Bodley Head. London. 1944.

ZIGMOND, D., *Scientific Psychiatry: Progress or Regress?* Update. October 1977, pp. 675–679.
ZIGMOND, D., *Transactional Analysis in Medical Practice.* Update. December 1977 pp. 1127–1137 and 1239–1241.
Personal View: an Anthology. British Medical Association. London. 1975.
The Future General Practitioner: Learning and Teaching. R.C.G.P. London. 1972.